It's Ok to Not Be Ok

Surviving and thriving while living successfully
with mental illness.

PRESENTED BY:

Kim LaMontagne, MBA

Perfect Time SHP Publishing

Published by Write the Book Now, an imprint of Perfect Time SHP LLC.

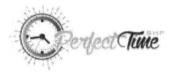

ISBN: 978-1-7329895-66

Table of Contents

Acknowledgements

I would like to thank my brave authors for bearing their soul. It has been quite a journey together and it has been an honor to lead you through this project. To my family – I love you! Thank you for your support and belief in me. To my amazing tribe of strong and impactful individuals around me – I love you all and appreciate your support!

To Jeff – The most kind, compassionate, easy going, supportive, strong and sensitive man. The universe sent you to me at the most unexpected time (7/28/2019 at 8:46 am to be exact) and in the most unexpected way. I am so grateful to have found you. I look forward to all our adventures together in Hope on wheels. Let's Go! I love you!

Foreword

One in five Canadians will experience mental health challenges at some point in their life. Either it will be something that lasts a short time or is more complex and is something a person will live with their entire life. This book being compiled by Kim is something that is needed in the world. Mental health is still seen as taboo, and not fully talked about in mainstream conversation. Here in Canada there is a day called Bell Let's Talk Day. A day where money is raised for mental health support across the country. Celebrities, such as actors/actresses, Olympic athletes, and singer/songwriters who live with mental health issues such as bipolar, anxiety, OCD, and depression are showcased all day on tv, radio, and social media about making mental health a topic we all discuss every day. Yet every day mental health is affecting many in the city I live, and I see it daily with those I interact with. We as a society need to talk about it more and be comfortable reaching out for help if we feel ourselves needing support with our own mental health challenges. I know for me I have reached out for help a few times to professionals and friends when I have struggled.

Kim is a Rockstar to be compiling this book, her care and compassion for the authors has been amazing to watch. It takes a lot of work to bring together so many authors in one space to share a vulnerable story. Kim answered everyone's questions, was patient with everyone, and encouraged every author to tell their story. Kim and I met through our coach Marlo Ellis from The Uncommon Woman. We formed a friendship and have remained good friends since we first took the course called Your 3 Minute Story back in February 2019.

I live with PTSD and high functioning anxiety. When I first tell people, I live with PTSD the most common response I get is "you weren't in the military?" And true, they are correct. Post Traumatic Stress Disorder is an abnormal reaction to a normal everyday event. My PTSD stems mostly from an abusive boyfriend who also stalked me at a university. I have been on the train that runs here in Calgary look up and see someone who for no fault of theirs triggers my PTSD. He may have a slight facial feature that reminds me of my ex boyfriend. Or I have been walking down a street and see ahead of me a man with a gym bag that has the logo and wording from my university, and that can also trigger my PTSD. I have also been triggered by a specific song I hear on the radio from time to time that was his favourite that we played a lot on the CD stereo at the university. I blank out, go numb, lose all colour in my face and stare into space.

I was at an event a year ago and a woman was sharing her story on the microphone. Her story was my story with a couple of differences. A friend who was with me and sitting at the table with me said that I started rocking and blanked out. It took my friend grabbing my hand and lightly squeezing it to bring me back to the room where we were at the event.

My anxiety is also tricky as it is high functioning. A trap of mine is catastrophizing, meaning I will over think negatively about a situation. For example, if I temporarily lose my ID I will think all the negative thoughts about how I will get it back, where did I leave it, and so on. It doesn't always look like a typical reaction to things that are triggering me. I will get anxious and fidget with my hands to help keep it low. I have been known to rock in my seat, laugh, create lists, or be busy with work, volunteering, and working on my business tasks to keep my anxiety at bay.

When I have no plans, my anxiety can creep up. There was a time not too long ago I was thinking about the first program I signed up with my coach, Marlo. At the same time my kitchen sink tap broke and I had an anxiety spike of how I am going to pay for both things. I couldn't think clear. I could tell that my anxiety was getting the best of me. I thought I should call a friend (I have a few I can call when my anxiety is spiking) yet I did not have the thoughts to know who to call. It took a lot of my energy to bring myself back to reality of being in my condo. After a while I was able to breathe, ground myself, and remind myself of the three things I see in the room, feel in my body (like my fingers typing on the keyboard right now as I type this), and three things I know to be true, like I am in Calgary, Alberta.

Within these pages you will read stories of overcoming adversity from women, and one amazing man! This is especially important because typically men do not talk about their feelings, or what is going on with them as easily as women do. I am proud of all the authors who have stepped up to share their personal stories of transformation. Stories of living with bipolar disorder, living with anxiety, living with an eating disorder, having suicide idealizations, and many more.

Every author has wisdom to share with you and wants you to overcome the challenges you may be facing. I know that inch by inch you can overcome the challenges you are struggling with. Reach out to us, the authors, Kim, or myself if you need support. We've all been there and done that. We've risen over our own mental health challenges and now want to help you!

Aime Hutton
International Best-Selling Author

Acknowledgments and Dedication

To those who feel their voices are not heard. We see and hear your silent voices. We will be the voice for you until you are able to share your story. I dedicate this to those who rise up over the ashes and inspire me daily. Special thank you to my coach Marlo Ellis for your support and guidance this year 2019. You have helped me be the woman I am today overcoming an anxiety fear that was crippling.

About Aime Hutton

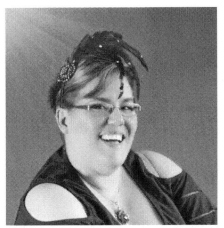

Aime is a true miracle survivor. Being born three months early was just the start of the challenges Aime has overcome in her lifetime. Hailing from Calgary, Alberta Canada, as a Girls Empowerment Leader, Aime empowers tween and teen girls to live their real brave selves full of happiness, courage, and confidence. She does this through training women to be Girls Empowerment Facilitators. A powerful program Aime developed over her 20+ years working with girls in a variety of modalities and her own personal development work she has done.

As a five-time international best-selling author/compiler Aime shares hope, healing, and inspiration through her writing. She was a finalist for the International Femtor Awards 2015 for eWomenNetwork in the category of Business Matchmaker from Dallas, Texas, USA. Being one of six in North America, and the only Canadian.

In 2017 Aime was awarded the Peace & Friendship Award by Diversity Magazine in Alberta for being one who celebrates, accepts, and learns from the Indigenous people of Canada.

e-mail: aime@inchbyinchempowerment.com

website: www.aimehutton.ca   www.inchbyinchempowerment.com

FaceBook: https://www.facebook.com/ibiempowerment/

Kim LaMontagne

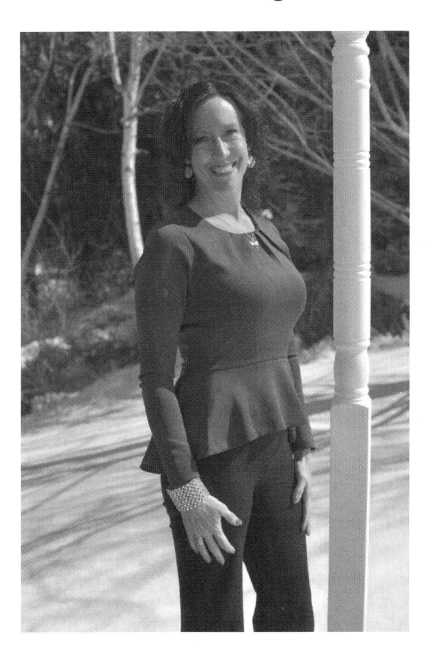

Introduction

Hope Anchored My Soul

Stripped…Raw…Brave and Courageous are four words to describe the authors in this book. Powerful, heart wrenching, hopeful and inspiring, describe the stories they share. I am incredibly proud of these passionate authors who have courageously taken off their masks to bring you this collection of stories.

Authors hail from across the United States, Canada and the United Kingdom. Each bares their soul and invites you into their world of darkness, recovery and hope.

Whether it's short term depression or a life of living with bipolar disorder, anxiety, depression, an eating disorder, substance use or suicidal tendencies - mental illness is life altering for the individual affected as well as the family.

Mental illness is an invisible disease clouded by discrimination, judgement, shame and fear. It is highly misunderstood. When experiencing the darkness of mental illness, sometimes what we need to move forward is to take that proverbial "first step." How does someone take the first step when they feel alone, ashamed, judged and with no guidance?

I offer these stories as your roadmap to help you or a loved one take that first step. These stories are meant to provide a 'light' for the person who is desperately trying to find their way out of the darkness and shame. Stories of strength and perseverance that give you or your loved one the most important ingredient in life - HOPE.

For the first 38 years of my life, I wore a mask to hide the guilt, shame and worthlessness I experienced as a result of being 'different'. I seemed happy and fun on the outside, but on the inside, I was empty, broken, jagged and on the verge of giving up.

Although I was on the verge of a breakdown, my performance in the corporate workplace never wavered. I have been a high achieving top performer in the workplace my entire life. On the outside, my high performance may have appeared seamless and effortless. On the inside, it was excruciatingly painful. I wore a mask to function at a high level. The mask hid the intense pain of the dark thoughts that were invading my mind every second of every day. It covered up the battlefield of a mind that was constantly at war with itself.

You're not worthy...you're not good enough...you don't deserve this life...people would be better off without you. These relentless negative thoughts were on replay in my mind 24/7. They were bullets of self-hatred that shot from my mind and pierced my soul. The mask also sheltered me from being exposed as someone with a drinking problem.

The mask was my armor.

I was a wine drinker. I drank 4-6+ glasses of wine every day to numb the pain. I was the life of the party and did some pretty hilarious things. I have experienced hangovers and many mornings with no recollection of what happened the night before. Two events stand out to me as complete reckless behavior.

After a sales meeting in Baltimore, I went out with a group of colleagues. I texted my then-husband to let him know I was going out and that I would text him when I got to my room. The next morning, I awoke to over 30 texts and phone calls from my husband, director and colleagues. I had gotten so drunk the night before that I don't remember getting back to my room and I never texted my husband. Overcome with fear, my husband found contact information for my colleagues on my company website and reached out to them. Everyone was worried! I overslept for my meeting and had a fight with my husband as soon as I woke up. I also had to explain to my director what happened. I played it off as a rough night.

There was a fire alarm in the hotel overnight. The entire hotel evacuated except me. I was passed out in my room. I wasn't aware of the fire alarm until my colleagues were discussing it the next day. Not my finest moment. I made it to the sales meeting and functioned the entire day. Everyone told me how funny I was the night before. I didn't recall a thing. Complete blackout.

I laughed along as they recalled the events from the night before. Behind the mask, I was riddled with guilt and shame and questioned my professional integrity. I was nauseous and sweaty all day. They served Mexican for lunch - Ugh.

Fourth of July 2009 was another fine moment. We had a neighborhood party at my house. It was a great time from what I can recall. When I awoke the next day, I was in my clothes from the night before. There were black marks all over my white pants. I asked my then-husband what they were from. I will never forget his response. He said, "Kim you were so drunk last night that you tripped and almost fell into the fire pit"! Hearing that was like a knife being plunged into my heart. My soul was bleeding. It was the exact moment I knew I had to make a change. Although my reckless behavior had never resulted in injury or harm to myself or others, I knew I needed to seek help.

On July 16, 2009, I made a phone call that changed my life. I called my Dr's office to make an appointment. I was finally ready to surrender and ask for the help I desperately needed. I called at 4:45 pm. Thirty minutes later at 5:15pm, I was met by the most compassionate, non-judgmental nurse practitioner I could have asked for. He held space for me that day. He saw me as a person first and not the disease. He saw me as someone who was suffering immensely with a manageable disease. He looked me straight into my eyes and said, "Kim - I am going to help you! We are going to do this together"!

His trust and belief in my ability to recover was exactly what I needed to make the pivotal change in my life.

On July 16, 2019, I celebrated 10 years of sobriety. Life is wonderful and so full of hope. Although I am no longer married, I have let go and fully embraced self-love. I have released all shame for my past behavior. Instead, I now see the reckless behavior as symptoms of the diseases I live with.

I have taken my pain story and turned it into power. By sharing my story, I have been able to reach thousands of individuals who also wear a mask to hide their suffering. Being vulnerable and honest with my struggles and recovery provides hope to so many who feel inadequate and shameful. It provides a safe space for individuals to know that I understand, and they are not alone.

My story is not unique. Many individuals suffer. What is unique is that I have the courage and bravery to take off the mask and speak my truth. As my coach Marlo Ellis says, be brave and stand on the shoulders of your story. That is exactly what I commit to doing. In doing so, I am providing hope to those who need it. Letting people know that - "It's Ok to Not Be Ok" and it's ok to ask for help.

To further support my commitment to spreading hope, I conduct speaking engagements across the country in addition to working a full-time corporate job. My goal with speaking is to share my story to reach individuals who still hide behind the mask. So many suffer in silence and are afraid to speak up.

I trust you will read these stories with an open mind and an open heart. It took an incredible amount of courage for these brave authors to step into this book project and speak up. They peeled back the layers of their story to share their truth with you. Bravery and courage defined!

About the cover

There is a special meaning and a subliminal image on the cover of this book. Butterflies are my favorite because they signify transformation. Upon embarking on this project, I hired Lori D'Agostino of Artworks by LBD to create a one of a kind painting to use as the cover. We discussed the color palate and the butterfly We also discussed using an image I had recently been given by Kristi Cornwell, Intuitive Business Consultant after an intuitive guided reading she conducted for me. At that time, I was searching for direction. Her reading was amazing. Many things she predicted have come to fruition. After the reading, Kristi texted me a picture and told me the guides told her to draw it. She did not know what the picture meant, but she wanted me to have it. Upon seeing the picture, I knew it was going to be part of something impactful. I shared the picture with Lori and she incorporated it into the background and butterfly wings.

Enjoy the beauty of her design.

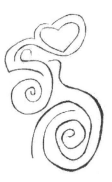

About Kim LaMontagne

Kim LaMontagne has devoted her life to helping others survive and thrive in the face of mental illness. After suffering in silence with anxiety, major depression, suicidal thoughts and alcohol use disorder, Kim has found recovery and a life of true happiness. A consistent top performer and winner of several Director's and Peer Choice Awards within her organization, Kim suffered alone in the workplace because of shame and fear of stigma.

Kim shares her story of recovery to help others find the courage, power and strength to rise above the fear, stigma and shame of mental illness. Kim is a Speaker, State Trainer, Teacher and Advocate with National Alliance on Mental Illness, New Hampshire chapter. She is also an Ambassador, Speaker and Member of the Advisory Board of Worth Living Mental Health, and a Member of the Dartmouth Hitchcock Health System Campaign to Combat Stigma and Discrimination in Behavioral Health. She is a contributing author to the book "The Strength of Our Anchors" and a Survivor.

She is a frequent speaker at conferences and conducts onsite workplace mental health presentations. She has written several blogs about mental health and contributes to multiple social media platforms to raise awareness. Kim believes we must start the conversation now about mental health. Especially in the workplace. Life is Worth Living.

Follow Kim on Facebook, LinkedIn and Instagram or contact her at Kim@kimlamontagne.net www.kimlamontagne.net

Cat Davis

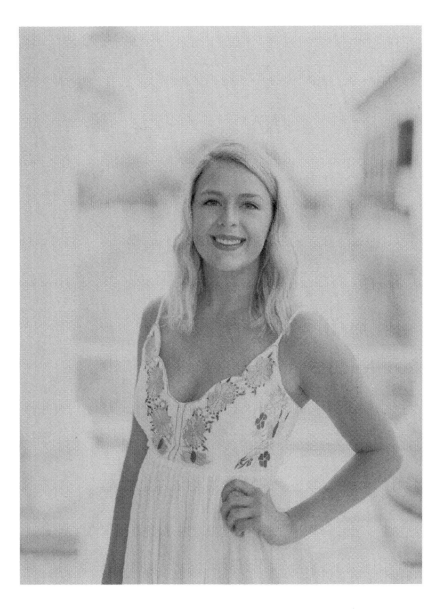

Locked Up

By Cat Davis

January 2017

They didn't have to sedate me. I went willingly. I had done this before, so I was numb to the process. Emotionally numb, no drugs needed. All I asked for were my own clothes.

"We have paper scrubs," they told me. "You can wear those."

But I did not want to wear paper scrubs. I did not want to look like a patient. I wanted to look like me, just a teeny tiny little bit like me if that was at all possible.

Eventually, they gave in and let my mom bring me a suitcase with some stuff from home. After a thorough examination, they let me keep most of it. But not my shoelaces. I had to walk through the impossibly clean, white halls with shoelace-less sneakers. If I hadn't been so numb I would have cared more.

I just didn't want to wear the damn paper scrubs.

I had been imprisoned inside my own mind for years, but this was the first time I was being physically held against my will. The first psychiatric hospital I was admitted into wasn't like this. I entered freely, and I left freely. Though I now walked in on my own two feet, I had no real choice in the matter.

The first hospital was set up like a single-story house with a kitchen and a home gym and a fireplace. There were eight perfectly petite bedrooms with twin beds and personal bathrooms and windows that didn't open and doors that didn't lock.

This second psychiatric hospital looked like... a hospital. There was a day room where the patients were to be confined from 8:00 am to 8:00 pm. There were a few puzzles and coloring books spread out on the tables, but most of the patients were staring blankly at a small TV in the corner. Across from the day room was a large desk behind which the nurses sat, watching the patients watch TV. The entire place smelled like bleach, and there wasn't so much as a smudge in sight.

I wasn't wearing shackles and I wasn't behind bars. But as I watched how meticulously the nurses unlocked and locked each door, I felt completely and totally trapped. It sunk in that I was stuck here until someone let me out. I gave up my freedom when I stepped through the doors of this facility. I was a patient, but more importantly, I was a prisoner.

I had no idea that I was about to be sentenced to life with bipolar, no parole.

* * * * *

Mental illness does not wait for the right time and place to present itself. It comes barreling through your life when you least expect it and attacks you relentlessly until you either bow down or go completely insane. I was 19 years old when I started making my rounds through mental institutions. I had to drop out of college to do so. What were supposed to be the happiest years of my life were being stripped away from me: classrooms were replaced with therapist offices; bars were replaced with pharmacy counters; friends and professors were replaced with fellow patients and psychiatrists. I became a deranged version of myself, rapidly switching from the highest of manias to the lowest of depressions. One moment I was insanely euphoric, on top of the world, conceited and completely enamored with myself. The next I was totally apathetic, incapable of pleasure, permanently exhausted and moving at an impossibly slow pace. Unlike unipolar depression, you are constantly fighting two battles with bipolar disorder (as the prefix "bi-" suggests). Rarely are you truly stable; oftentimes you are just riding the waves. Up and down and up and down.

I do not believe the opposite of happiness is sadness. I do not believe the opposite of happiness is hatred. I believe the opposite of happiness is simply numbness. Numbness is an all-encompassing feeling that derives from intense psychological pain. It shuts down your mind, allowing you to passively continue on with your day without falling to pieces. Numbness is your body kicking into survival mode after experiencing pain.

Though what your body doesn't know is that this very emotion meant to save your life might end it.

* * * * *

TRIGGER WARNING: SELF-HARM AND SUICIDE

January 2012

Numbness is what led me to start cutting. Slicing my wrists, and then slicing other body parts, open with broken razor blades. Numbness is what led me to two suicide attempts, the first one when I was only 14 years old.

A recent breakup had left me feeling completely and utterly hopeless. The absolute agony of losing him was too much to handle. Numbness swallowed my body; it engulfed my soul. The frantic mess I felt suddenly turned into immense calm. I quietly, thoroughly searched my room for pills. I swallowed handfuls at a time: Advil, Melatonin, Midol. And I waited.

I fell asleep.

And I woke up.

Passively noting my obvious non-deadness, I got out of bed. I put on my school uniform, grabbed my backpack, and headed out to my first-period class.

And that was that.

* * * * *

June 2013

I didn't see a therapist until I was 16 years old. I told her about the cutting. I told her about the numbness. I told her about the pills. I told her many things over the course of our six months together. None of it made a difference. She didn't think anything was wrong with me. She worked primarily in social work, and couldn't identify any root causes of my problems. No trauma, no abuse, no violence, no neglect, no poverty. Nothing. There was nothing that she could point to in my past that explained my present negative moods and self-harming behaviors. So she listened patiently to everything I told her and then determined that nothing was wrong with me.

And that was that.

* * * * *

November 2016

I realized that I was bipolar three months before I was diagnosed. I was misdiagnosed with depression at the time, and I was taking an antidepressant that was rapidly and ferociously tearing me apart. The antidepressant attempted to diminish my depressive symptoms by forcing serotonin to stay in my brain for longer than it typically would. Unfortunately, and unbeknownst to me at the time, many people diagnosed with bipolar experience severe adverse reactions to this increase in serotonin, including the triggering of a manic episode.

And yet, no one realized that I was experiencing mania. Not the doctors, not the therapists, not even me.

Until I did. I knew that I wasn't getting better on my antidepressant. In fact, I knew I was getting worse. Desperate to find the answers the professionals weren't giving me, I started researching my symptoms—all my symptoms, not just my depressive ones—online. I came across a description of bipolar disorder, and I found myself mentally checking off boxes in my head, especially as I read about mania. Racing thoughts? Check. Grandiosity? Check. Psychomotor agitation, racing thoughts, impulsive and risky behavior? Check, check, check. Examining the symptoms of mania and depression side by side, I knew I had figured out what was so wrong with me.

My psychiatrist promptly dismissed my concerns. She told me that I was not bipolar and that I didn't want to be.

Obviously bipolar did not ask for her or my opinion.

* * * * *

January 2017

I had seen twelve therapists and four psychiatrists by the time I was admitted into my second psychiatric institution. Receiving treatment at my first hospital felt almost like a fluke; after some soul searching, I was able to half-convince myself that anyone could be hospitalized, not just the most abnormal, unfixable members of the human race. Upon entering the second hospital, I quickly came to the conclusion that I *was* in fact the abnormal, the unfixable, and that was why I was locked up not once, but *twice*. I had gone from a freak accident to a frequent flyer. I figured the bleached walls and fluorescent lights were my new normal, and any fight I had left in me faded away. I didn't even care about seeing the hospital psychiatrist the next day. I figured he would just tell me the same thing everyone else had: that I was depressed, end of story. After poking at some hard pasta and taking my nightly meds, I peacefully fell asleep without so much as a single tear.

Believe it or not, being diagnosed with bipolar disorder was the highlight of my time locked up. Don't get me wrong; the competition for second place in there wasn't very steep. But what for some people sounds a death sentence sounded to me like a resurrection. My fifth psychiatrist heard me, believed me. He pronounced me bipolar and saved me. The numbness melted away, replaced by the slightest bit of tingling sensation throughout my body. Feeling. I was feeling again. Finally, I was feeling again.

With the newfound knowledge of my bipolar disorder came great responsibility. My psychiatrist told me he would not release me from "crazy people jail" until I had a plan *on the outside*. I needed a full mental illness maintenance crew: doctors and therapists and constant "support" (my friends and family). My antidepressant was replaced with two new fun pills: a mood stabilizer and an antipsychotic. *Yikes.*

The word "psychotic" freaked me out at first; that is, until my therapist helped me realize that I had actually experienced psychosis many times throughout my life. I had experienced both hallucinations—false sensory perceptions—and delusions—false beliefs—before and after I was diagnosed.

I had once hallucinated that I saw a long-gone ex-boyfriend at my gym. And that I had seen my dead grandmother at the foot of my bed. But the most severe psychotic episode I had was a hallucination-delusion combo conjured up by my brain when I was 16, while I was under the care of my very first therapist.

* * * * *

November 2013

I went to the bathroom, but when I stood up, all I saw was red. Blood. Lots of it. And something big and hard that had sunk to the bottom.

I sat down on my bed, head in my hands, contemplating what I had just seen. I felt sick. I knew in my gut what it was. My boyfriend had visited me a month or so earlier. It had to be. I knew it was.

I was pregnant. Or I had been pregnant. I felt it. I thought it. I knew it. I had just had a miscarriage.

I called my boyfriend sobbing. I didn't know what to do; I was so sick and so sad; I had just lost a baby. I knew I had. He cried too. He believed me. He knew it was true too. I thanked God we had each other to get through this. I knew I wouldn't be able to handle it otherwise.

I didn't tell my parents anything; they didn't know I'd ever even had S-E-X before. Except one day I couldn't help it—my hormones must still have been out of whack or something. I started sobbing while my dad was dropping me off at school and I told him the truth: that I had been pregnant, but I had lost the baby. I held my still bloated stomach, and I ached. My dad didn't know what to do; he certainly wasn't expecting the confession. He just held me.

The first few weeks were the hardest. I wrote a lot, more than I had in a long time, penning many poems about our baby. My boyfriend and I named her Elizabeth, my middle name. We cried constantly. But we knew we could get through this because we could get through everything. Because we had each other.

This was a shortened version of one of my poems (which I still had saved in my phone six years later):

Mommy isn't really a mommy

And daddy is just known as a man

But we both love you

We know we're your parents

You're just in another Father's hands.

We cry because we miss you

We're sorry we had to let you go

But God has better plans for all of us

And you were too perfect, we know.

Big colored eyes

And olive toned skin

And fattened cheeks smiling ear to ear.

My baby is healthy

My baby is perfect

Too perfect for life down here

For Elizabeth.

It doesn't get more real than that, does it?

Except it does.

Because my mind made the whole thing up. The blood was a hallucination, the pregnancy, a delusion. But the emotions, the torment, the life-altering, soul-crushing heartbreak: that was all real.

I silently carried the weight of this delusion with me for years until I finally recognized that it was not real, it never had been real, and it never would be real. With this realization, I was finally able to overcome the delusion's grasp on me and let it go. But not without the gut-wrenchingly horrible knowledge that I wasn't the only one whose life had been irreversibly marred by a figment of my imagination.

All I can say is that I'm sorry, that I didn't mean to, that didn't know my mind could play such terrible tricks. But I can't even bring myself to say that.

I hope and pray the hallucinations and delusions never come back. Even though I know that, if they haven't already, they probably will.

* * * * *

Present Day

I am scared every day that I will relapse. I am worried that my meds will stop working. I am terrified that I will have to be locked back up in a hospital, that I will become so numb again that I will have no other option. I worry about becoming pregnant—for real this time—about becoming a mother, about holding a steady job and maintaining a stable marriage. I am only 22 years old, and yet I think of this not-so-distant future constantly.

But I persist. I write. I speak. I listen. I comfort. I do these things because I want to, but more importantly, because I have to. I have to believe that my bipolar disorder is here for a reason: that I am here for a reason. I was locked up for years in my own numbness, in my own insanity, but now I feel. I cope. I understand.

I am free.

About Cat Davis

Cat Davis is a 22-year-old student at the University of Virginia studying Cognitive Science with a concentration in Neuroscience. As an advocate for mental health awareness, Cat has shared her own experiences through speaking platforms such as TEDx and The Human Library Organization. She is the Director of Worth Living USA at worthliving.co, a global initiative that allows people to contribute to the conversation on mental illness through their writings, podcasts, music, and artwork. She has also published articles on iam1in4.com, selfgrowth.com, mental-health.alltop.com, and her blog highrisk1.wordpress.com. Cat aspires to publish a memoir about her time navigating two psychiatric facilities at only 19 years old before being diagnosed with bipolar disorder. She hopes to educate the public about the signs and symptoms of bipolar disorder and advocate for the research of mental illnesses, which she believes will inevitably lead to more correct diagnoses.

Follow Cat on LinkedIn, Instagram, Twitter, Facebook, and her blog! Let her know that you found her through "It's Ok to Not Be Ok"!

Blog: highrisk1.wordpress.com

LinkedIn: linkedin.com/in/cat-davis/

Instagram: @highrisk1   Twitter: @highrisk1cat   Facebook: High Risk 1 by Cat

Dedication

I proudly dedicate my chapter…

To my family: Mom, Dad, Hunter, Momo, Grandad, Aunt Lizzie, PauPau

To my healthcare providers: Dr. Anderson, Anonymous

To my professors at: Baylor School, University of Virginia

To my hospital visitors/shoulders to cry on: Ally, Jess, Natalie, Grace H, Grace D, Sara, Meghan, Kelly, Katie, Haley, Sam, Lauren, Ariana, Cam, Andrea, Nicole, Molly, Brennan, Anna S

To my personal editors: Anna L, Maddie

To my homegrown friends: Sophia, Catey May, KB, Lane, Presley, RayRay

To my high school friends: Emily, Sarah, Stella, Katie, Kate, Mary Claire, Bella

To my friends abroad: Adam, Iain, and the rest of Fountainbridge Pres

To Worth Living:

I could not be more serious when I say that I would not be alive without you all. You saved my life when I was at my darkest and continue to give me a reason to live at my brightest. Thank you.

Cat Davis

Keeley Winfield

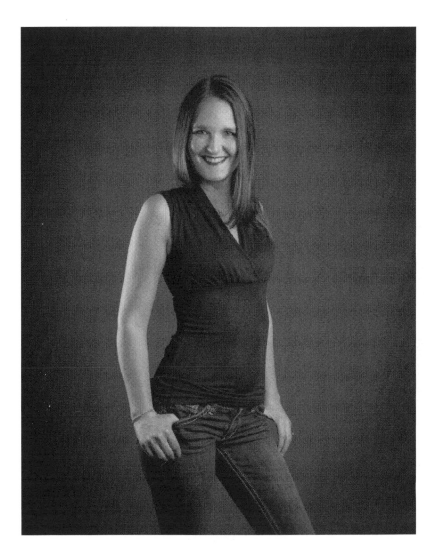

Moving Forward with Grief

By Keeley Winfield

I grew up in a normal middle-class household. We had a minivan, a cat, lived in the suburbs and I went to public school. I was eight when my parents separated. While the separation and divorce were hard on us, my dad has always been a huge part of my life. He moved just up the street from us and I loved being able to walk between their homes. My parents did return to being friends and talked at least weekly.

When I was seventeen, my childhood home went into foreclosure in the market crash; my mom moved in with her boyfriend while my older sister and I moved into an apartment. One night while driving home, I was hit by someone quickly changing lanes, so hard that my car instantly stopped running. I didn't have time to break before she hit me, it happened so fast! My beautiful silver Honda that I purchased myself was totaled and I was devastated. I moved in with my mom and her boyfriend until I could get a car. I was working full-time; life was normal and good. Or so I thought.

What I didn't know was that my mother was suffering from depression and addiction. I didn't know the signs. I was at work that October day in 2010. I was nineteen. My mother called me and asked when I would be home, she was crying. I asked if she was okay and told her I loved her. Just a few hours later, while I was alone in the office, her boyfriend called me crying. He told me that I needed a ride home, not to drive myself, and to come home right away. I demanded he tell me why. After trying to avoid answering, he said "You mother killed herself. I'm so sorry. Come home." I dropped the phone and fell to my knees. I let out a primal scream. I called my friends who had just left the office and asked them to come back. They did. I couldn't bear to be alone. I don't know what I would have done without them sitting there with me while I waited. I don't remember anything they said, just them being there I'll never forget. Shock.

I called my cousin and told him not to tell anyone. I didn't think it was true. I thought she was pranking me for not spending enough time with her. He hurried over to take me out there. I don't remember the drive there. Only a moment of staring out the window wondering what I was about to go home and see. Denial.

It's all a blur. When I arrived home, there were police everywhere, in the front yard, all over the house and they wouldn't let me go upstairs. I had to identify her because her boyfriend wasn't family. I don't remember leaving the house or getting back to my car. I don't remember when I went back to the house, where I slept that first night, or if I even slept at all. Shock.

We planned the funeral, all a blur. I wore her favorite dress she bought me, green, brown and strapless. Numb. I didn't cry at the funeral. We had it in a hotel conference room and so many people came, we had to open a second room. I've estimated around two-hundred-fifty people. Friends and family went up and spoke about her. So many people loved her and always described her as the woman who could light up any room with her blonde hair, sweet demeanor, and loud and infectious laugh. Options were there. She didn't see them. I kept expecting her to walk through the door or the phone to ring. Denial.

I went back to work before the funeral. I ran out of a group interview, that I was running, hysterically crying. I was so deep in grief that I couldn't fake happy. How could I fake happy when I felt so angry at her! I couldn't believe that she would leave us like that! I was snapping and blowing up on people. Even snapping at my boss once, which lead me to being fired as an assistant manager. Deep shame. Drinking too much. Staying at different houses to avoid being home where she died. Dating men who weren't good for me. All toxic. Hating myself for not seeing it. All a blur. All numb. A cycle of emotions I didn't understand and couldn't name. Anger.

I found her stash of pills in a locked box in her closet the police hadn't found. One-hundred-nine pills, opiates and muscle relaxers. I thought if I took them, I'd somehow understand. Somehow this was all a dream and she would come back. I kept trying to pick up the phone to call her and then would remember. I started to obsess over how one change here or there could have saved her life.

Had she just told her therapist what was really happening. Had I called someone when she called me crying. Had I just left work. I could have made more of an effort to connect with her and really see what was happening. We weren't ever taught about the signs of depression, mental illness, and addiction. Just a week or so before her death, she was holding her baby picture and asked me "Why did no one love this little girl?" Why didn't I see how big of a red flag that was? Any number of things could have changed it, but I didn't know and I didn't see it. Bargaining.

About two months after her death, I moved into my own apartment. I took the pills with me. Continued seeing men who treated me terribly, moved onto buying pills when the pills ran out, and I stayed numb. I felt more energy with the pills. I made more tips serving tables when I took them. One day I forgot them, went to work without one and had my first withdrawal. I knew enough about addiction at that point to know what that meant. I had to stop. I quit cold turkey and cut ties with people who I knew had them. Some people felt abandoned during this time and didn't know why I cut ties. I felt ashamed. Like somehow, they were stronger than me. That's when it all sunk in. I was no longer numbed. I had to feel it. I remember lying on the hardwood floor in my bedroom crying. I didn't feel worthy of the bed. In that moment I thought, "This is it. I either get up and pull it together, or I'm going to end my life. I cannot live like this anymore." I thought about my dad and my sister and all they had been through. Depression.

I reached out for help. I had a friend who was clergy in a Pagan church and she referred me to a friend of hers. He met with me for free in his church every week for a couple of months. I slowly started to pick myself up. I quit my job and got a better one with health insurance. I started to work on my self-worth and self-love. I still struggled, but progress was happening. I went back to college, I started to look for men who would treat me right and someone I could see a future with. I made a list of all the things I wanted in a man and surrendered it to the universe. I found new friends with positive mindsets who wanted to help lift me up. I put up boundaries around people that I felt were still in habits I no longer wanted to be part of. Those boundaries allowed me to love them without them pulling me back into the old place I didn't want to be. Testing.

The truth is that I'll never be okay with how she died. I'll never be okay with the millions of things that could have gone even a little bit different to result in a different outcome. I place no blame. I understand that suicide is an act of great anguish and hers had no singular "cause". Now it's up to me to heal. To heal myself, to heal the wounds that are left behind, and to share my story to help others. It took me seven years after her death to start talking about it. Once I did, I found healing through sharing. Acceptance. Grief is tricky. Many people have heard of the five or seven stages of grief, but rarely do we discuss that they don't always go in order. Each stage can be revisited several times in the process. I condensed the story here, but this whole process happened over two years and I wouldn't say it's complete even now. I revisited each stage over and over again. Grief is like a sticky web that pulls us back in again and again. We don't "get over it" and we don't "move on." We move forward with the grief; with the people we lost. Their life, loss and what they meant to us will always be a part of who we are. My mother is still a voice in my head, a love within me, and a wound on my heart. She will forever be a large piece of me. We move forward, together.

I've learned to understand masks. Masks we wear to hide who we really are and what we're really feeling. We all have masks. That mask we use to hide the hard times. The mask we wear to seem tough when we feel weak. I refuse to do that anymore. I don't believe in weak. Showing emotion is strong. Healing our wounds is strong. Crying is strong. Grieving and moving forward with grief is strong. If that means I cry in public, then so be it. I'd rather live as authentically me as I can, be vulnerable, and give others permission to be vulnerable too. Brene Brown says, "There is no courage without vulnerability."

I learned about stories. The stories that we write around our experiences. The stories we tell ourselves about situations and things that haven't even happened yet. I found that there's the story we tell about what happened and there's the story of what really happened. We create meanings in things even if there is none. Our minds take in so much information every day that they have to edit the information for our conscious minds to process. These filters form the story and the memory. Memories aren't a screenshot of an event; they're deleted, distorted, and generalized stories around an event. That's why two people witnessing one event can have completely different stories or memories about what happened.

I do not believe that everything happens for a reason. I believe that everything is the outcome of an infinite number of free choice decisions and every decision we make has an infinite number of outcomes and ripple effects that we may never see. I find this comforting. If I do my very best every day, I can touch lives far beyond what I can see. Because of this, I can find a silver lining, a lesson, and a place I can grow in everything I do. I try to do that. I don't believe that my mother was "supposed" to go through depression, anguish, addiction, misery, and die by suicide. I do believe that I had a choice with how my life could go following that and I've chosen to let that pain, that period of not being okay, fuel me towards helping others and preventing suicide. It's pushed me into sharing my story to help others see the aftermath of someone dying of suicide. The heartbreak, the anguish, the pain, and the not being okay.

I also believe that every happy moment, smile, laugh, movie, holiday, and Saturday mornings eating orange rolls also shaped me, grew me, stretched me, and contributed to my ability to see the silver linings. At least that's my current story.

Talking about what happened has been massively healing for me. Releasing the shame I felt around it. Being around people who could understand my pain and weren't afraid to talk about it. Reading books, listening to audio books, listening to podcasts, and learning about healing, mental illness, addiction, and people overcoming hardship was revolutionary for me. Finding people who could love and support me through my struggle was lifesaving and life changing. I found meditation, journaling, music, support, NLP, EFT, hypnosis, community, and more that helped me get to a place of love and acceptance. A place where I can tell my story, hear your story and it's no longer a deeply painful trigger. It's a place of pure love, compassion, and empathy. We can all heal. We can all hold unconditional space for each other with no judgement, no advice, and just listening. We can hold each other up when we're falling down, or fall down together and hold each other there, so long as we're connected.

I will continue to teach the tools that helped me most, to fight for better, more accessible mental health services and better options for people to get help. But for now, it is okay not to be okay. We will all not be okay at some point in our lives. We will all grieve something! We all know someone who isn't okay. When we band together and accept this, accept that it's okay not to be okay, accept that we can be here and be a space through someone else's not okay-ness, then we will see less deaths. We will save lives. We are never alone in our pain. We are never alone in our thoughts. We are never the only one feeling this way. There is always someone out there who is willing to be a space and to listen. You're never alone because we're all in this together.

I dream of a world where we have community and a village. A place where we're working together to support each other, to raise our children, to heal, to love, and to feel supported. I believe humans are pack animals and we're seeing a spike in illness because we all feel alone and without the pack. This is something we can fix, together, no one has to be alone. It's up to us to heal, to reach a place we feel healed and whole enough to hold each other, to be vulnerable and open, to trust, and be sure we don't bleed our wounds on people who didn't hurt us. I personally choose to still be open, vulnerable, and hold others while I heal. Healing together. I hurt other people in my process of healing. It's okay not to be okay, and we're still responsible for our words and actions. Let's heal together and show others that it's possible too.

Acknowledgements and Dedication

I would like to thank my husband for always supporting me and being patient with me in my chaos of new projects!

I would like to thank my sister for always loving and supporting me! And for helping me edit my chapter!

Big thank you to my father for his humor in hard times, his unconditional love, and for never turning away from me.

To my beautiful, fabulous friends, family, and village, I love you, more than I can put into words! Thank you for always being there, even if I disappear for 7 weeks to write a book and take back to back courses!

To my fellow authors, thank you for your great bravery, vulnerability, and authenticity! The world is a better place for it!

About Keeley Winfield

Keeley Winfield is a loving mother of two, a wife, a coach, and an advocate. Her mother's death by suicide, as well as surviving other painful tragedies, has sparked her journey towards healing, growth, and renewal. As an advocate for mental health and suicide prevention, she is dedicated to holding the space for conversations around these, and many other difficult stigmatized topics. Always learning and exploring new concepts, Keeley actively seeks additional training and resources, such as being an NLP master practitioner, so that she can best support those around her in learning that "it's ok to not be ok."

Keeley is on a mission of self-love, discovery, and finding more enjoyment in such a chaotic world. As a life coach, speaker, and writer, she is always encouraging others to share their stories and to explore those stories in a safe, productive way.

Megan Harmony Franko

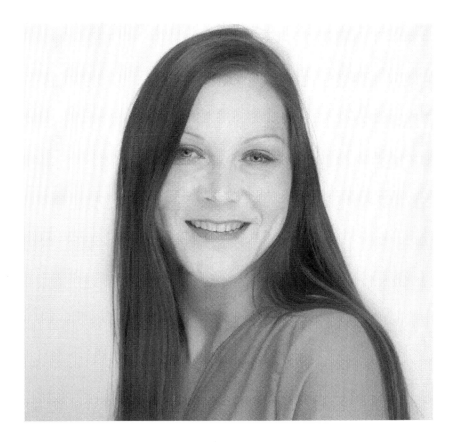

The Puzzle Piece That Is Me

By Megan Harmony Franko

When I was a little girl, I had big dreams and aspirations. I knew I was meant to change lives. Maybe my larger than life personality comes from the fact I am a Leo Zodiac. Maybe all kids get super excited when a camera gets pointed at them. While this was my reality and I was a happy kid, I also had a deep knowing that I was different. I experienced the world in immense ways. I loved to sing and was quite the talker in my toddler years. I learned things pretty quickly when taught and I really loved life. In grade three, I even received a certificate for being third in the province for math. I loved math. I felt everything very deeply. The world didn't always make sense to me but I made the best of figuring it out. I organized my dresses from shortest to longest in my closet and my shoes were always matched up. I studied people to try to understand my surroundings. I went to church and loved to swim. The care bears was my favourite show and every member of my family can recite all of the worlds to 'Labyrinth' and 'The Princess Bride'. We watched them on repeat because of me. When I was interested in something, I devoted all my time, energy and effort towards it. My parents sometimes would take one shoe as a joke but that REALLY stressed me out. My parents divorced when I was four. Around that time, I was diagnosed with juvenile diabetes and started on insulin injections.

In grade seven, I went through what many young girls do. My *so called* friends were mean girls and wanted to be my friend one day and made fun of me the next. I would receive notes saying my hair wasn't clean and my clothes were dirty. I didn't understand how friends could act this way. It didn't make sense to me. My lifelong toxic love affair with excoriation disorder (skin picking) started at this time while I was trying to process the overwhelming emotions of these experiences. One day I couldn't take it anymore. I felt worthless and unlovable so I ran to the bathroom. I sat in the stall with a notebook and wrote my will. 'I leave my dog to my Mom and my stereo to my Dad'. In that moment, I made a decision that I was going home to end my life. Then there was a knock on the stall. "Are you ok?" A voice rang out. Another girl in the class had seen me run off with tears in my eyes and she saved me. We became the best of friends. I thank God for her often.

On the last day of grade nine, I picked up my English exam and I had scored 69/70. Someone called me a "goody two shoes brown noser" and I decided to show them. I proceeded to get drunk and high that night and this started my 11 year battle with alcoholism and addiction. Substances helped me to fit in and subdued the confusion I often felt. I was able to be a part of life (sort of). The worry thoughts would stop temporarily when I took the first shot, toke or line. Eventually, it turned on me and stopped working. I was too far gone by that point to stop on my own.

At the age of 18, life was going ok. I moved out of my home because of a fight with my mother. She told me to get out of her house. I took that as a literal statement because I saw the world based in facts and black and white. When she said it, I listened. I came home one day to get my suitcases for the basketball tournament I was headed to and my stepfather and I had a lovely conversation. This made me very happy because he struggled with severe, can't get out of bed depression. On this day he was very chipper and seemed at peace. I went for dinner with a friend, my stepfather said he would grab the suitcases out of the attic for me. When I returned later, something felt off and the suitcases weren't out. Then the phone rang "Honey, it's Mom, you need to come to the hospital right away." My stepfather had attempted to end his life and was in critical condition. He remained in the hospital for three days and then passed on. I was shattered as I had been the last one to see him alive and talking. I blamed myself and took ownership for many years. My substance abuse increased at this point. I needed more to numb the pain, thoughts and guilt.

I entered into a romantic relationship which was messy because of our substance abuse. At the same time, the relationship provided comfort. He really got me. Up until this point, I hadn't felt that anyone had. I was always the odd one in the group. I never felt like I belonged. I knew I was different from other people and I struggled to do the day to day tasks required of healthy living. Eat three meals a day, do the dishes each night. Anything that required organization was increasingly difficult for me. I turned to hoarding behaviours after my stepfather's passing. I literally kept everything. This young man in my life, was strong in the areas I struggled with and we brought a beautiful baby girl into the world. She was my saving grace in so many ways and makes me proud every single day.

Things started to improve but the substance abuse came back with a vengeance once she stopped feeding from me. At this time, I had a great career, the love of my life, a beautiful young daughter and a nice home. Things seem to be going pretty well, but I was struggling and then things shifted in our home. We fought a lot, separated a few times and then finally decided to end it.

At this point, I was completely lost. I had set quite a few rules for myself related to love. 'When you love someone when's it time to call it quits? Never!' 'True love lasts forever.' 'When you love someone you stay together forever and it's happily ever after. These rules came out of the movies I watched as a kid because I learn how to live in this world based on what I see and experience around me. So this break up didn't make sense because it didn't follow the rules.

I spiraled downhill fast. I chased men trying to find my forever love. A pit of despair and loneliness like nothing I had ever known before. I was taken to the hospital by ambulance due to low blood sugar after drinking. I had to take sick leave from work because the pressures of everyday life were too much for me to handle and my face from the picking was an awful mess. By this time, I had turned to using tweezers on the spots to get out the 'pus' that was in there. I was getting infections on my face and so desperately wanted to stop. It was the only relief from the overwhelming emotions I didn't know how to control. My problems were piling up on me. I would forget to a pay a bill or I would spend the bill money on substances instead. My house was a mess. Things were just getting worse and worse and I had no idea how to improve my life. I resigned myself to the fact that I, in fact, just suck at living life and was incapable of doing better. I had tried so many ways and nothing was working. I always ended back in a disaster of one form or another. People were always mad at me for the things I said. I just couldn't live life successfully.

At the age of 26, my parents came to my home to find me projectile vomiting in my bathroom due to high blood sugar. My father took my very worried daughter to daycare and my mother drove me to emerge. My heart stopped while there and they had to revive me. I hadn't taken any bolus insulin in ten days. I didn't realize it then, but I was trying to put a stop to the insanity that was my life in a way that wouldn't cause my loved ones the pain I had felt at 18 because they would believe my diabetes caused it.

A few months later, I started my sober journey and life began to improve. I really started to get my life back together. My daughter trusted me and knew I was going to be where I said I would be. I obtained full-time employment at my job. My family and friends no longer worried they would get that call. I had money in the bank and my bills were being paid. My face even healed with a few scars but I looked good. I met and fell in love with a great guy who met my high list of standards. Everything was going great. Although I still struggled with social interactions, things were good.

A few years later, things took a turn with my partner. I found myself in a situation that I didn't expect. I wasn't sure what to do. He was still using substances. We had a home together and were raising "our" kids. I suffered an injury at work that left me unable to work. My daughter started being bullied and suffered with her own mental health concerns. Life started to get hard again. The relationship dissolved and I couldn't go back to my career. Finances were dwindling. The thing about me is, when life is going well, I am able to manage day to day tasks. When things get stressful or hard, I tend to shut down and curl up into a ball. I was finding myself on social media for hours at a time. I would just disconnect from the real world and live vicariously through other people. I knew I needed help so I turned to the people who had helped before. Although I hadn't picked up any substances, life had become increasingly difficult. I called the woman who had been my sponsor a few years previous. She works the 12-step program as outlined in the big book. I got back into the work. Things improved but there was still something off. I asked my doctor to send me for specific mental health testing to see if what I had felt for a few years was true.

After a yearlong wait, the assessment was done and I was diagnosed with Autism Spectrum Disorder, Excoriation Disorder and Major Depressive Disorder (in remission). I was 35. At the time when the doctor said this, it felt like the gates of hell had clanged down on me. *"YA! Great - I have an answer to why life has always been so difficult but in the same sense I'm not normal."* I felt like I would never understand other people and my business idea to help people would never work now. Luckily, I have an incredible support system, who I leaned into at this time. They reminded me that this is an answer to why I have had so many problems. The diagnosis was actually a solution. I was told that this gives me an advantage in business because I am a No BS coach. I tell it like it is. I am able to notice things that other people might not catch and share it from the heart.

Things people said to me when I shared my diagnosis include, "You don't look autistic", "That seems to be the new fad diagnosis these days, doesn't it?", "REALLY, you?". I want to challenge these things by saying the tag line for autism 'You know one person with autism you know one person with autism.' We are all unique in what our strengths and amazing abilities are, as well as unique deficits. It is not a fad diagnosis. They are just realizing the deficits that didn't used to be present in diagnostic criteria and more people are being appropriately diagnosed. For the most part, people were very supportive and said, "That makes sense." This diagnosis for me was a God send. I no longer feel like an outsider in this world. I'm not an alien. Now, I understand that I don't have to state every fact that enters my mind. I've learned that not everyone thinks and behaves the same as me. The areas where I used to be vulnerable - oversharing when first meeting new people, trusting that everyone is good intentioned are less of a struggle. Not everyone is always telling the truth and just because I am a truth teller and truth seeker, does not mean that everyone else lives this way. The world and its people are less complicated and it is possible to live an amazing life as a person with autism. This does not mean everything goes great all the time. I have my high functioning days where I face life for the most part successfully. Then there are the days where I have been overstimulated or have an awkward social interaction and life feels dauntingly hard. Overall though, I'm learning and growing and never lose sight of the hope that carried me through all the years that I knew I was different but didn't know why. Hope and love carried me through the darkness back to my soul where there's an abundance of light.

I know that for me personally, I need a strong connection with my Higher Power to help me navigate through life. A strong tribe of incredible people to be there when things get tough. A support system of passionate individuals who hold space for me on the days where I want to give up. This is essential to living life soulfully. I now spend my days helping others face challenges. I am a healer. My Reiki treatments and coaching are changing lives. I share my story on stages and have a podcast as well. My experiences led me to a place of sharing that IT IS possible to have an amazing life no matter what is happening around you or what diagnosis you have.

Never give up, never lose hope, better days await you. I became a hope dealer and inspire others to find hope in the darkest of places. You deserve an epic life! Believe that.

I was a puzzle piece trying to fit into a puzzle I didn't belong in. Now I have found my home. It started with loving myself enough to know that the answers were out there and (to continue) seeking them.

I figured out the puzzle piece that is me.

Acknowledgements and Dedication

I want to thank my beautiful daughter Trinity for being my greatest teacher, as well as a supporter when I struggle. My sister for helping me navigate through life especially when things were difficult. My Mother who has come to my rescue on many occasions and helped me through the chaos. I want to thank my Father and Step-mother for their encouragement and support.

Thank-you to my dear friend Holly who has stuck by me since high school and helped carry me through the storms and heartaches. Thank you God for always being there.

Thank-you to the Canadian Mental Health System, I wouldn't be where I am without the help I have received. My various tribes for their ongoing love and support when all felt lost. Words can't begin to express the gratitude I have for each of you and everyone else who has crossed my path.

Thank-you

About Megan Harmony Franko

Megan Harmony is the founder of Soulful Sobriety, it's not just a community it's a lifestyle. Megan is passionate that IT IS possible to live an incredible life, even when the you know what hits the fan. She is a champion at rising above the ashes whenever tragedy or heartache come into her life and has the ability to heal people through her words, presence and skills. Megan believes that love is a universal language everyone understands and devotes her life to spreading hope everywhere she possibly can. She will ignite the flame within you, when you feel it has flickered out and reminds us that each day we get to choose what our day will be like. Megan wants to leave everyone Soul Full having met her and can't wait to meet others soul to soul.

Megan is an inspirational speaker, a healer, an author and brings out the potential in her clients. She creates the space for them to let go of the baggage they have been carrying around and start to believe in themselves. She helps people thrive through adversity and stay sober through it all. She teaches how to live life loving yourself, feeling worthy and excited for each new day.

Her lived experience, Master Level Arcturian Reiki and Light Healing Practitioner Certification, Practical Nurse Diploma, and Addictions Careworker Diploma make her uniquely qualified to assist people through their most difficult times.

To understand Megan's journey to sobriety in more depth, read her chapter in The Great Canadian Woman Book available on Amazon.

IG: @soulful_sobriety | FB: @MeganHarmonyTLC Podcast: The Soul Full Podcast with Megan Harmony available on most podcast players.

Wendy Sterling

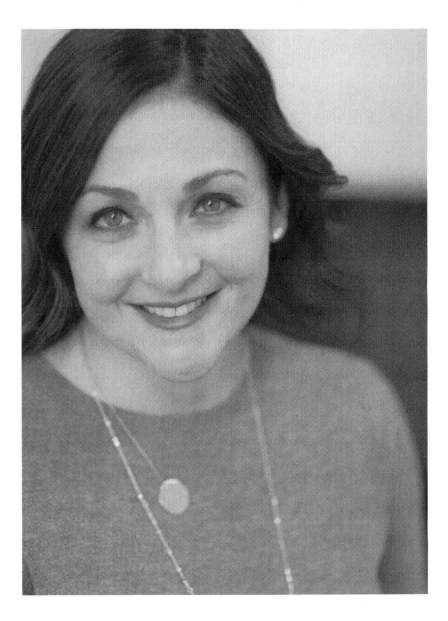

Divorce Has A Silver Lining

By Wendy Sterling

I am in our bedroom searching on his iPad. Staring back at me is a naked, graphic picture of his much younger co-worker. She is professing her love and obsession for him. The "him" is my husband. My husband. I collapse onto the floor in shock, tears streaming down my face, unable to catch a breath . . . My stomach starts to churn and fill with acid, burning my insides, rage slowly building in my head. I take the iPad and throw it against the wall. My intuition is dead on. I wish it wasn't.

My husband is having an affair.

It was August 2016 and I remember it was a warm, summer night. We were driving home from dinner with another couple when his cell rang. It was *her*. A young production assistant who he worked with. I looked at the clock and it said 11:45pm. He sent the call to voicemail as quickly as he could. I stared at him and asked, "Why is she calling you this late?" A pain shot into my stomach when he immediately dismissed my question. She called again. And again he declined the call. My breathing sped up and my heart started pounding. I glanced back at him and asked "What does she want from you this late at night?" He explained she probably got into a fight with her boyfriend and wants to vent. I silently looked out the window and thought to myself *why would he be her first phone call? Don't girls call their other girlfriends first?* We sat in silence the rest of the way home, my head and thoughts spinning in circles.

When we got home, I marched down the hall to our bedroom, while he paid the babysitter and walked her out. He came into the bedroom and my instincts took over. The next voice I heard was my own, saying "Give me your phone." His reaction was immediate. "No!" I was startled and taken aback. His story was that she got into a fight with her boyfriend, and he was the only one able to talk both of them off the ledge. Why him? The wheels in my mind were churning. What was really going on between them? In that moment I knew there was something inappropriate about their relationship… but until now, I never had a reason to doubt his love for me. He was the *last* husband who would cheat – that was everyone's perception. Yet right then and there I knew he was *exactly* that guy. When my husband came back into the room ten minutes later, I continued asking over and over for him to give me his phone. He kept refusing, telling me it was fine and he handled it. Rage started boiling inside of me. It was a feeling I had never felt before. He was hiding something. In fifteen years we had never gone to bed angry. Until that night. I was furious and terrified of what my gut was screaming at me.

The next morning at the gym, I replayed the night before over and over in my mind. It was a merry-go-round I could not stop. Why was *she* calling my husband so late at night? Why wouldn't he give me his phone? What didn't he want me to know? As his wife, I have a right to, don't I? Either way I knew I had to confront him, and I was determined to get answers the moment I got home.

I walked in the door and sent our two boys, 10 and 6, upstairs to play. I looked my husband dead in the eye, and my tone made it clear that this was a demand, not an ask. "Give me your phone… *now*." He not only again refused, but manipulated the issue back on to me, questioning why I was still talking about last night. My insides were on fire, boiling and about to burst. I cried and screamed that I was not crazy. I started to shake with fear and became so overwhelmed with rage. With betrayal. With shame. Trust was gone. My heart was breaking. My boys. Our family. I became numb. My best friend for the last twenty two years was a stranger. Next I heard a voice scream, "Get the fuck out of my house, you son of a bitch." And I realized that voice was me. As he left, I crumpled to the floor in tears, convulsing until I got on the phone with my best friend. The first words out of my mouth were "I just kicked him out."

My husband and I had been in couples therapy for the last two years, trying to learn how to communicate better with one another. Ironically, we had our weekly standing appointment the next day, and agreed to keep it. Hours before, I was standing in our bedroom and glanced over at his nightstand. He left his iPad behind. I immediately picked it up. A voice told me to open it and search for emails and text messages from *her*. I so badly wanted to be wrong. I wasn't.

There it was. It was shocking, sickening, and overwhelming. I discovered years--literally *years*--of emails, messages, pictures, and so much more. The volume was too much to comprehend. My feet gave out from underneath me and I slammed onto the floor, crying a puddle of tears until our appointment.

We sat on opposite ends of the couch. My purse clutched to my waist with the iPad inside. Our therapist sat across from us in her chair. The room was dimmed. I remember looking out the window, at the tall buildings, the blue sky, wondering if this was real. Or was it a dream? Do I have the strength and courage to confront him? I want my husband back. My family back. I wanted to erase the other night. For the first time in any of our sessions, I sat silently, unable to speak. Words escaped me. Instead, my face and swollen eyes said it all.

He initially denied all of my accusations in front of our therapist, and justified his inappropriate friendship with *her*. Mid-sentence, I reached into my purse and pulled out his iPad. I choked out the words, "I think you forgot this." His face went ghost white. My hands started trembling and tears rolled down my cheeks. Having already queued up the most graphic and telling email of them all, I started reading it out loud. He froze. Words were coming out of my mouth, but they were his words to *her*. Not mine. Words and emotions I always dreamt he would say to me.

From that moment forward, his excuses kept coming. Not a day has passed where he has ever attempted to share the full truth with me. Sure, he gave me versions that paint him in the best light, even going as far as to portray himself as the victim. I know I will never truly know everything, but the extensive information I did find was enough to file for divorce.

My marriage was officially over.

I sunk into the deep depths of my mind and a depression I still don't know how I managed to get out from underneath. My family life on Facebook appeared "perfect" and we were the last couple this would happen to. He was the *last* person to cheat. The embarrassment and shame were overwhelming. I thought it was my fault. I lost my appetite and could barely function enough to get my kids to school. I cried in the car. I wished I could run. Leave him behind. I wanted someone to wake me up from what felt like hell. How did this happen to me? WHY did this happen to me? How did I not see this? How stupidly blind was I? I trusted him. I believed in him. In us. In our dreams. Supported his career. Supported his late work nights. Believed the boys and I were his world and he would never do *anything* to jeopardize it.

I stared at the empty pillow next to me each morning, which brought instant tears. Making breakfast, packing lunches felt like insurmountable tasks. For the first time in my life, I was caring for my boys as a single parent. And then there was my new job, which I started *one week* after I caught him cheating. So, I threw myself into work. Faked a smile and pretended to be happy. I snuck into the bathroom to cry. I worked out a lot. I lost 15 pounds in two months. On my 125lb frame I was the smallest I'd ever been in my adult life. Looking in the mirror, I didn't recognize myself. I had dark bags under my eyes, pasty white skin, dry hair, a thin frame and a dark cloud over my head that only I could see. No appetite except for what became my nightly two glasses of wine and chocolate. Those closest to me knew I was slipping away.

I couldn't keep up the charade much longer. I was barely hanging on. I knew an intervention was needed, but didn't know how to ask for help or where to start. I was not good at asking for help and saw it as a weakness. I believed I was strong enough to do this on my own. I couldn't let anyone think I was unable to manage all of this. What would they think? I didn't want anyone to think I was weak or that we were having marital problems. I always figured it out. I am a problem solver. Why should this be any different? I knew deep down this was one time I could not do it alone. I had to ask for help. For me AND for my kids.

One day I was looking in my bathroom mirror staring at my reflection . . . and I had NO idea who she was. Someone who lost her way, fell off her path, sacrificed so much, was unhappy, lost faith and craved more in life. Where did you go? How did you get so lost? Looking at myself under a microscope felt awful; yet at the same time, it felt oddly freeing. I knew it was *exactly* what I needed to do. I already shed more tears than I knew possible by one person. Exhaustion and sleep deprivation were becoming the norm. I lived in a fog. A fog of denial and it was not working. I knew I had to take a step towards finding a piece of myself again.

But I wasn't ready to ask for help just yet. Instead, I started doing Google searches for books I could read. I typed in key words like depression, shame, guilt, trust. What I found stunned me. There were authors, researchers and women like me who understood what I needed to hear, to help me see so much I never knew or learned. To face the parts of me that needed to change. Growing up, I did not understand that sharing your feelings and being vulnerable was a strength. I believed in God, but didn't understand what trusting the universe meant. I was mesmerized and craved to read and know more. These women provided me with so many gifts and self realizations through their words - and it was just the beginning for me!

TRUTH ALERT!

I failed in parts of my marriage. I did not honor who I was or what I wanted. I saw happiness in the reflection of my husband. I lost my voice. My identity. Seeing this for the first time made me want to fight harder to find myself. I thought if I threw myself into more self-help books, my new job and raising my boys, I would get there. Regardless, I felt like the real me was still hiding, afraid of what I might discover. There was a pull towards needing more of something. I didn't know what that "something" was, until a friend's Facebook post appeared in my feed. She left her law degree behind to become a life coach. My gut and intuition told me to call her ASAP.

After our 3-hour call, which included a lot of tears, laughter and coaching (which I didn't know at the time), I knew becoming a *life coach* was my new destiny. To help others, and to mentor and help guide them towards a better path. I immediately enrolled in the courses, and little did I know, my entire life was about to change.

Without those courses, classmates and instructors, I know I would not be where I am today. The incredible part of the program is you not only learn *how* to be a coach, but you work on *yourself* at the same time.

For the first time I was able to bring my own dark thoughts and emotions into a room full of strangers. The ones I hid from my closest friends and family. Those thoughts I hadn't shared with anyone else. The tears I only allowed myself to cry in private. I finally found a way to be true to myself about what I was discovering and who I wanted to become. I learned so much. What I wanted. What I wouldn't tolerate. What is important to *me*. And who I never want to be again. It was like the foggy glasses I wore for decades were suddenly wiped clean. I failed myself. Shame on me. But guess what - it was *okay*.

It is about what you do **after** the failure that counts.

Failing means there is a lesson. With lessons come learning. Through learning comes growth. From that moment on I vowed to change. For me. For my kids. I finally found the catalyst I needed to heal the pain of my divorce and look ahead. Coaching. And along with that came a judgement-free, safe place to feel what I needed to among a community who were once strangers and became my closest friends.

Therapy, books, doctors, friends – I tried it all, but nothing had the impact on me as life coaching did. I knew that the universe had a larger, better plan in store for me. It took my husband cheating on me to see it. To see the silver lining that my divorce was a gift. The gift of finding myself. Gaining back my self-esteem and confidence. Building an even stronger version of me. Finding peace. Using my voice. Learning to genuinely smile. Seeing the lessons in everything.

It's not about who I would still be if I stayed married. It is about who I *wouldn't be* if I hadn't left him.

I followed my heart and rebooted my career as a *Divorce Recovery Strategist*, where I use tough love to help divorced women end their pity party, mourn their marriage and MOVE ON with dignity to see that life is better afterwards!

Acknowledgements and Dedication

Adam Sterling
Sam Sterling
Max "The Bernedoodle" Sterling
Mom and Dad (Rosa and Fred Suessmann)
Betina and Adam Baumgarten
Stephanie and Adam Zaffos
Gregory Poppen
My Amazing Besties Squad (Janet, Traci, Mirissa, Cathleen, Arin, Kelly)
Leah and Matt Emerick
Evan Pinchuk
Dr. Sharon Schwartz
Tracey Thorsen
Marlo Lyons
Co-Active Training Institute (CTI)
My CTI Classmates
My Find Your Light House Tribe
My Journey Forward Tribe
My Accountability Buddies
My Coaches (Krista, Jessica, Kelly)
My Angels (Emma and Anthony)
The Universe

About Wendy Sterling

Establishing her career as a top-level advertising sales executive in the digital space, at the world's most progressive social and lifestyle website brands (such as *Who What Wear* and *Refinery29*), Wendy Sterling had it all... successful career, two beautiful children, and a (seemingly) devoted husband. But after enduring a traumatic and unexpected divorce along with her mother's cancer diagnosis, Wendy's entire world was rocked to its core. It was in that dark moment when she decided to screw the "poor me" attitude, and allow her sass to emerge alongside her class.

Leveraging decades of experience as a mentor, problem-solver and strategic thinker, Wendy followed her heart and rebooted her career. After becoming a CPCC and ACC certified coach, she transformed her mission into being a *Divorce Recovery Specialist* with the goal of helping divorced women boost their confidence and sense of self, while releasing their guilt, anger and fear. Wendy provides a tough-love approach using her successful, first and only *Divorce Rehab*™ program, alongside the community she's built, to move countless women through the pain of their divorce quickly. Unlike other divorce coaching programs out there, her program was developed using the steps she used after her own divorce.

Wendy currently lives in Los Angeles with her two boys and dog, Max. Connect with Wendy via email at wendy@wendysterling.net and on Facebook and Instagram (@youtwopointo).

Emily Nuttall

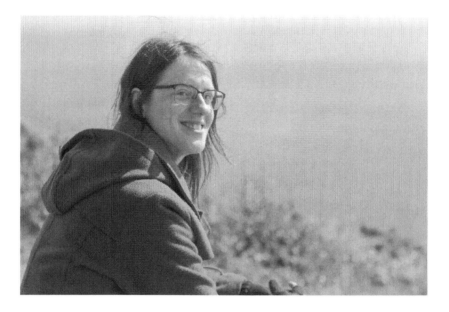

Behind the Mask

By Emily Nuttall

I was born on September 4, 1993, in the Princess Elizabeth Hospital in Guernsey, in the Channel Islands. I was an only child. In my early childhood years, I would have loved to have a sister to play with. She would have long, blonde, curly hair and blue eyes, just like Alice in Wonderland. I imagined brushing and playing with her hair, dressing up in princess costumes, pretending we lived in a big palace with pink and purple walls, butterflies, fairies and golden staircases. Unfortunately, so early in my childhood years, this was something I could only dream about.

I guess all expectant mothers; think about all the amazing things to come. They plan for their due date hoping that everything will be okay with their baby's all-round development. Sadly, sometimes unexpected things happen, and new family life must temporarily be put on hold.

When I arrived into this world, I had other ideas than my mum did. I wasn't going to be a patient baby and wait happily inside my mum's warm, safe tummy until my due date. Instead, at 24 weeks into my mother's pregnancy, my mother's water broke. I arrived eight weeks early, weighing in at only 4lbs 4oz.

After my early entrance into this world, the professionals decided I needed to spend a short amount of time in an incubator in the special care baby unit. What an adventure this was, to lie in a rectangular box with machines beeping and wires all over me. Totally unaware of what was happening, I had a great time in the incubator. I was an angel for the midwives, liking all the drama. But on the other side of the incubator, my mum, dad and other family members were filled with anxiety.

After a period of time, I was strong enough and healthy enough to come out of the special care baby unit.

If you are prepared enough for your baby's arrival, you may have read all kinds of books to try and help understand what to expect over the many months and years ahead. You may have come to understand what age your baby will reach its key milestones of sitting up unaided, rolling around, crawling and finally walking and talking.

But me being the stubborn, mischievous baby that I was, I didn't want to make life easy for my mum and dad. I was not meeting these milestones as I should have been. After months of a range of different tests, doctors and surgeon appointments, x-rays and scans, I was diagnosed with cerebral palsy at 12 months old.

Cerebral palsy is a condition in which physical movement and development are negatively affected as a result of damage to the developing brain, during pregnancy or just after birth.

By the age of three, I became aware of what was happening and was fascinated by it. I watched my mum and family putting these intriguing splints on my legs, followed by funny looking boots, then giving me bright yellow coloured children's walking sticks. Having found my newfound freedom meant I became a tiny tearaway and always up to mischief.

September 11, 2001, breaking news hit us of the 9/11 terror attack in America. Whilst thousands of people stayed glued to their television screens, I was being prepared for one of the most terrifying days of my life: operation day. I brought my favourite teddy bear, it was pink, soft and fluffy, and it came to all of my treatments with me. But I was still afraid.

As I was getting prepared for surgery, I acted strong, brave and confident for my family. Daddy told me I was his brave little girl. I watched my surgeon and all the other professionals surrounding my bed, with their surgical masks, aprons and gloves. They talked through everything with me, reassuring me that I was safe and that it would all be okay. After this brief discussion, they took my family aside to go through the final pieces of paperwork.

Suddenly the strong, determined, smiling nine-year-old with all the confidence in the world let down her brave face. Fear finally consumed me. I was scared and in pain. I was no longer ready to face what was ahead of me. Sobbing into my pink teddy bear, I felt confused and lost.

To admit to pain and fear would mean that I was weak, or even worse - ungrateful. After all, I was being offered life-changing surgery, which I knew would ultimately improve my life. On operation day, I learnt how to put on my mask of confidence.

It was the end of October 2001, I went back to school, it was a bright autumn day, leaves were falling from the trees onto the school playing fields. I was walking with my sticks with my bright pink plaster cast visible. I had been fortunate enough that my cerebral palsy had not affected my intellectual development, which I was grateful for. This meant I could attend mainstream school with extra support. On this day, some boys from my year group came up to me. They were much taller than me. One of them had a big build and spiky hair. His big booming voice screamed at me that I was stupid, ugly and fat. He pushed at me, whilst the other boys laughed, jeered and encouraged him.

I felt rejected, judged, isolated and lost. But I couldn't show I was afraid because I didn't want to be a further target. To feel safe and protected, I kept my mask of confidence close to me. I just wanted to feel accepted. At the end of the day, I was still Emily. Since operation day, I had always kept my mask of confidence close to me. After the boys tormented me, I put that mask on. I knew I couldn't let me fear defeat me, so I had to rise above them. I spoke to my teachers, and with some extra help and support, the bullying stopped for a good period of time.

Facing cerebral palsy has thrown all kinds of hurdles at me. I suddenly lost sight in my left eye in 2005 and in 2010, I was diagnosed with scoliosis. These physical challenges brought much uncertainty into my life. I felt fearful, lonely and isolated. With my mask of confidence, I was safe. Using my mask, I didn't let other people's judgements affect me.

I still face many challenges with my cerebral palsy but I realize that being fearful is okay. I'm in a place now where I do not let fear overpower me. I face every life challenge with confidence, determination, strength and hope because "when you fear your struggles, your struggles consume you. When you face your struggles, you overcome them."

December 13, 2008, my world came crashing down around me. My gran suffered a sudden stroke and died after five days in the hospital. I was at my dad's house. He sat me down in the conservatory. He came down to my level, put his hand on my knee and looked into my eyes. I knew she was gone.

I felt it was my fault that she suddenly died, just before my gran had suffered from her stroke, I had gone to her house. I wasn't coping with what had already been two years of a devastating, painful and frightening family breakdown at my dad's and I took out my frustration on her.

My dad divorced my mum when I was three years old. I had always been a daddy's girl, but he found a new partner who became my stepmother from day one. I was not accepted into her family. I always remember her dark black hair and scary eyes, and the look on her face. Full of rage and evilness, when she would emotionally abuse me she would scream at me that I was worthless, ugly, fat, a failure and a mistake. That I had ruined her family. She would isolate me from my other siblings by keeping me in another room in the house. When I would visit, I would witness shouting, arguing and terrifying violence between her and my dad. It made my dad's house feel at times like a war zone.

My relationship between my birth mother had also broken. We were always fighting and I struggled to get along with her boyfriend. I felt like a lost teenager trapped and at a crossroads, not knowing which way to turn. This made me more angry and broken. By this point in my life, family support services had become involved. They had intervened one year earlier, desperate to keep the family together to stop everything collapsing into a big wall around me. But it didn't work.

On the last day I ever visited my grans house, I was overwhelmed by distressing flashbacks, emotional pain, sadness and fear. It felt like a washing machine on spin cycle, going around constantly inside my head. I was a scared teenager and didn't know how to communicate my distress. I screamed at my gran at the top of my lungs that I hated her, everyone and everything and wished I was dead. I told her I wish she and everyone would go away forever. These were my final words to her before her stroke and death.

In the three years prior I had started fighting a silent battle with my mental health. Wearing the mask of 'I'm fine' guarded me from the pain. It helped me go numb, forget everything and be strong for everyone around me.

But underneath this mask, there was so much more: depression, anxiety, self-harm, suicidal thoughts and anorexia. It had consumed my mind and body. When I was younger, I had imaginary friends. Someone I could talk to, play with and give me a sense of belonging. They were there for me through the difficult things happening in my life, keeping me safe and helping me to cope. My 'I'm fine' mask became my new best friend.

January 2015, on a cold winter's day, I was asked to come to my doctor's office for my anorexia and thoughts of suicide. I waited anxiously in the waiting room, my mind and body had finally given up the fight. My hands and feet were blue, cold and numb. My eyes were sunken, my body gave up functioning, and my hair fell out in clumps every time I touched it. I felt disconnected from everything around me. My doctor entered the room, took one look into my frightened eyes, and saw beneath my 'I'm fine' mask. She saw that I was weak, exhausted and broken. My heart pounded violently in my chest from anxiety as my general practitioner (GP) called the mental health inpatient unit. After hearing her umm and ahh, she carefully put the phone back on charge. She put her soft, warm hands onto my painfully bony shoulders, took my hand and calmly said, ``I'm sorry, but I have to send you back to the inpatient unit.''

Tears quickly filled my tired eyes as I begged for one more chance to go home. I promised I would start to eat and drink again and keep myself safe. I wasn't going to the inpatient unit willingly. Anorexia, depression, self-harm were my best friends and I couldn't lose them. In my distorted, fuzzy head, I was still a fat, ugly, worthless piece of shit and I didn't deserve to be alive.

I had no choice. The ambulance drew up outside, followed by paramedics and the police. I had finally admitted defeat. I was sectioned under the mental health act, which meant I was forced under the police and doctor's orders to be admitted back to the inpatient unit. I was handcuffed to a police officer and wheeled out to the waiting ambulance. With the flashing of the blue lights, the wailing of the sirens, I was taken back to the mental health unit.

Living under this mask of 'I'm fine' made me feel guilt and shame, which made asking for help so much harder. I was broken and I was hurting, listening to my best friend, anorexia I restricted my food constantly punishing my body. The physical pain I felt every time I did not allow myself food numbed my emotions and gave me respite from the vicious war in my head. I needed and deserved to be punished; I was ashamed of Emily. I hated being stuck in my own mind and body, but at the same time it felt safer and easier not to open up and let other people see my despair.

Having been such an angry teenager, I couldn't show this again. Instead, I was angry at Emily. Since I had never felt in control of my body due to my disabilities, surgery, emotional abuse and bullying, I could punish it instead. I wanted my mind, body and soul to fade away to be free and at peace. The 'I'm fine' mask destroyed my mind, body and soul.

For so long, I let myself believe the lies of anorexia and the 'I'm fine' mask. The I'm fine mask made me a liar; it made me hate my life and everyone around me. It made me cry; it made me break and wanted me to believe I was a mistake.

I realise now that I can't allow it to take me over anymore. I am the only one with the right support and determination to be able to get my life back on track. I know I have to be brave, honest and strong enough to reach out like the old Emily needed and wanted to. I have to show the mask that had been my best friend that I know it is in fact a nasty bitch that wanted to kill me.

I'm still on the journey of recovery, which feels like a roller-coaster full of ups, downs, twists, turns, loopdaloops and backwards drops. "Healing is never a straightforward path". There are times now where I'm tempted to pick up the I'm fine mask to protect myself, keep myself safe and helps me to cope when I am struggling. But for me it's a dangerous path, a slippery slope, taking me back to a dark and scary place. I've had to trust myself as Emily, be honest with people, accept myself and be proud of Emily for being so determined to create a positive, healthy future and help encourage others to be brave enough to break free of their masks.

Because behind my mask is a breaking heart, a mind and body that's falling apart, a face that shares a story of strength and hope, that through the struggle there is a better way to cope. The light at the end of the tunnel is somewhere in sight it will be a hard battle, but worth the fight.

Acknowledgements and Dedication

I would like to acknowledge the following people for helping make this possible:

Kim Bolton LaMontage- for helping me, inspiring and encouraging me with my chapter

Cat Davis- for helping me with editing on my chapter and for also encouraging me as a person

Steph Bisson- my amazing website developer for the use of photographs and for doing these for me

Louise Vivian- for being there for me, guiding me and supporting me

Beat Eating Disorders- for providing me with support, leaflets and information for the book and supporting me with the media releases

To my family and friends that have stuck by me through this journey and my continued recovery with my anorexia, mental health and disabilities thank you for being there, believing in me and for never giving up on me

To all my doctors, surgeons, physiotherapists, my eating disorder and mental health teams and other charities including Beat, Mind and Action for Children thank you for continuing to support me and for giving me so much strength and hope everyday with my continued recovery and treatment.

I dedicate this book to all those struggling with Disabilities, Mental Health and Eating Disorders, you're not alone. Have hope, believe and never give up.

All proceeds from the sale of my book will be donated to Beat Eating Disorders who continue to help and support me with my ongoing recovery from anorexia

About Emily Nuttall

This is a true story, of how Emily Nuttall has overcome adversity and wants to inspire others to be able to do the same. Emily was diagnosed with cerebral palsy at 12 months old, has suffered a detached retina in her left eye at the age of 11 and is a survivor of emotional abuse.

At 16 Emily was diagnosed with scoliosis. From the age of 12 Emily has faced significant mental health challenges including anxiety, anorexia, depression, autism and suicidal thoughts. Emily is on a journey in life one where she has worn a variety of masks, to hide behind, to protect herself and others and to help find her sense of belonging in society. Removing these masks Emily is now revealing the strong but at times vulnerable woman beneath who continues to fight on her road to recovery and to one day fully break free.

Emily works as a volunteer, speaker, coach, champion and campaigner to create a positive and healthy future for her and others. Emily's story will share her journey of what lies underneath these masks and how she is now breaking free and fighting back on her recovery journey, helping and inspiring others to do the same, break down stigmas that surround mental health, eating disorders, youth homelessness, suicide and disabilities.

To hear more of Emily's story please visit emilynuttall.com which will be coming soon. You can also connect with Emily and hear more of her work and story on Twitter @emily4993 or Facebook Emily Nuttall.

Jeffrey E. Berger

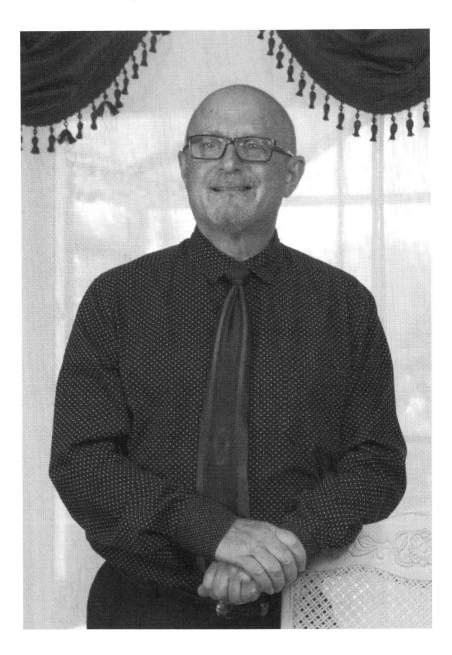

Rocking The Boat On My Journey To Mental Wellness

By Jeffrey E. Berger

It is only recently I started to come to terms with my own personal journey. Over the past 55 years, I'd been hiding deep down behind male macho bullshit. The Catholic guilt was there because of so many years of teachings embedded in my being from an early age. For as long as I can remember, I instilled in myself, "Build a bridge and get over it!" This statement has haunted me in so many ways. It didn't allow me to feel, express my emotions or certainly not be the real me. I have forever stripped that out of my consciousness, apologizing to those I've hurt with my coping mechanism for so many years. It has led me to a special attention to developing more compassion for others.

It all started in December 1964; I was ten years old. My family moved to a small-town outside Buffalo, New York.. The new school system, new surroundings, new people and thoughts of I'm a creep started to emerge. I knew something deep down was very different. I couldn't figure out what it was. For years, I kept thinking, what the hell is wrong with me? I didn't know how to describe it, nor would I ever attempt to talk about those feelings with anyone. I didn't fit in! I was petrified.

This is when I recall my internal, dark struggles started. I was challenged daily to understand who I was... More like what I was. I just didn't know anyone else who had similar feelings. I felt people were talking about me. The looks and teasing from my peers tormented me. It was so excruciating that I just didn't want to be around anymore. It was even more difficult competing with my identical twin brother who was not "that" way. Patterns that would haunt me over the next ten years were now emerging. I was afraid of saying, "I'm okay." How could I when I was so different.

I remember wanting to study piano in the fourth grade. I found the perfect escape over the next several years, advancing quickly with a new instructor. It was during my mid-teens when the sexual abuse started. He sat next to me on the piano bench. It progressed to his body pressed against mine. The actual piano sessions started to get shorter. We moved into his private back office with small talk and him showing me naked pictures. Finally, instead of my hands on the keys, his hands were moving up and down my thighs. "It's okay, that's what men do", so I thought.

He demanded I never tell anyone because it was private and it was no one else's business. It was the perfect time to lure a fresh, young, naive and introverted kid into the lion's den, enlisting in mutual trust and secrecy. That's how it always starts. The abuse continued for a couple of years. I was so afraid I couldn't find a way out. I just couldn't tell my parents; I didn't want to disappoint them and was afraid it was my fault. I am gay.

It was 1973. High school graduation and time for my initial flight to freedom; off to college I went. We'd just come out of the sex, drugs, and rock n roll hippy days of the Sixties. A new era was emerging. I'd grown up as a gay teen and was now entering what would become the more sophisticated, sex, drugs, and disco days. Its hallmarks were big, puffy, sprayed hair, tight bell-bottom pants, platform shoes and so much more. I was just coming to terms, or so I thought, with who I really was. I still wasn't out of the proverbial closet. This is when I noticed a more pronounced onset of severe stressors, anxiety, depression, and my initial, serious suicidal thoughts. It was a constant, ongoing, internal daily battle, having to hide who I was for fear of being rejected, humiliated and even outcast by family and friends.

In May 1974, I returned home from my first year at college in West Virginia. Eighteen was still the legal drinking age and I was desperate to find my first gay bar. I remember like it was yesterday. I parked away from the bar on a side street so no one would see my car. Walking to the bar I was scared shitless looking around to see if anyone was watching me.

I walked down those few steps into the Hibachi Room, "Don't Rock the Boat" was the song I heard, entering my first gay bar and seeing all these men on the dance floor. I felt I was home. It was exhilarating seeing and being around people who were just like me. It gave me an initial sense of comfort. Thinking back, now I laugh.

Later that same summer, I entered my first male relationship. I had no idea it would turn into one of the most traumatic, mentally and physically abusive relationships I'd ever have. It continued for the next several years as I still hadn't come out of the closet. My boyfriend always had to be the center of attention. He had to know where I was, what I was doing, and who I was talking to at all times. I wanted out so bad, yet again, I couldn't.

A third man was introduced, forming a small, intimate lounge band. We started playing locally, eventually taking to the road up and down the east coast between New York and Florida. Performing allowed me to escape into my own little world not having to deal with reality. I put on a great act those years pretending on the outside everything was perfect, when deep inside I was crying for a way out. Still, I couldn't find the courage to come out to my family after hearing so many stories of friends who were disowned. I felt completely trapped not having the courage to leave my relationship because I was threatened with exposure to my family.

The days turned into weeks, then months, and finally years. My state of mind grew worse until one night I totally exploded. The anger and rage built up from several years reaching its final limit. I still clearly recall lashing out, attacking him, bringing him to the ground, taking his head in my hands and bashing it into the cement walkway.

I wanted the bastard dead. It took the other band member who was more than six feet tall, which seemed like hours to pull me off. My hands were wrapped around my boyfriend's head like a vice. I was determined. I wanted him gone. Period!

After being pulled off, I literally snapped. My adrenaline was thrashing inside my veins, my body so enraged I didn't want to go on with my life. If not him, me. I was so sick of my life; I didn't want to live this way anymore. In a split second, the decision was made. I ran down the hall through the apartment, stumbling into the bathroom. I locked the door. My hands were trembling. I took a razor blade to my wrists. Scared out of my wits and at the same time trying to understand what was happening. Just then, my bandmate kicked down the door and wrestled me to the floor. I failed at the attempt.

Today I look back and just thank God. It was a short time later I finally had the courage to leave what was the most horrific relationship I'd ever had. I still hadn't shared my true self with my family – not even my twin. It was time to move onto new and better things.

It was the early Eighties when the AIDS crisis started. It just seemed to get worse and worse. Living in an age when it was common to be called "Faggot," "Queer," and "Sissy," these names only compounded my ongoing internal struggles. I remember walking down the street, minding my own business when cars would drive by with a group of immature guys yelling gay vulgarities, and throwing bottles sometimes causing bodily harm. Just living with the stigma made day-to-day life humiliating and demoralizing. The media made constant reference to AIDS as the "gay disease." Religious fanatics and homophobes made sure to tell us it was God's way of punishing us. I thought I had it bad before, but the thrashing, internal, mental torture continued with so much negativity from the media and society lashing out at the gay community.

I had to get out; I wasn't happy. My only way was to escape to somewhere else, anywhere away from where I was. I wanted to be in an environment where I could start to be the real me. Being around other gay people gave me a sense of self-worth.

I moved to New York City in September 1984 with $14 dollars in my pocket. It's what artists did to pursue the big dream. It was both the best time and a very terrifying next chapter. I got sucked into a deep, very dark subculture: The Saint, Underground, Mine Shaft and the Limelight were the places to escape to, a world of pure ecstasy. Why? Because that was one of my party favors. These clubs allowed me to fully enter into a fantasy where nothing was wrong but also knowing there was a tremendous risk. I found it exciting, mind-blowing even. I truly felt accepted, or so I thought. I remember wanting so much to be liked, loved and accepted, but being a part of this culture came with a price then, unfortunately for all the wrong reasons.

It was early 1985 that I was savagely raped by someone twice my size. I was pinned down thinking horrible thoughts of being sodomized and left for dead. Fortunately, that was not the case. However, for the next six to nine months I endured more anguish. Even worse than the physical pain. This came from having to wait for blood tests after the fear of AIDS exposure as my rape was unprotected. I would stay busy to eliminate any thoughts of what the outcome might really be. But when I arrived home at the end of the day, the thoughts raced through my mind with outbursts of crying and lots of praying. Thank God my results came back negative. I was so grateful to retain my good health.

My life consisted of working full-time, performing with the NYC Jazz Company, auditioning and living a wild nightlife. I worked hard and partied harder. On the outside, it seemed like I had it all. However, the darkness inside continued with self-doubt, extremely low self-esteem and severe depression. I was crawling and sprinting through an incredibly fast-paced life in the city that never sleeps. Sometimes I went directly to work from the clubs, then rehearsals and performances. It all took its toll on me emotionally, physically and mentally. I kept pushing through it all, being tough, continuing to say "I won't fail; I can't fail" because that wasn't me as it would have simply destroyed me.

My time in the Big Apple came to an abrupt halt due to an injury sustained performing in a rock video. It ultimately provided me an opportunity to leave the city that I so loved. I believed it was my message from God, telling me it was time to move on. I was looking forward to a new change escaping the high-risk lifestyle. Or so I thought.

In January 1988, my move to Boston was a fresh start. New life, new city, new people and looking forward to leaving all those memories in New York. Although my passion was still in the arts, entering the corporate world seemed to have its own excitement. I had new opportunities since completing a software technology program at Columbia University. I was fortunate to secure a position with one of the top software companies in the world.

Unfortunately, I relapsed into severe depression ultimately leading me back to substance abuse which was the only way I knew how to cope through extended years of depression and low self-worth. It was excruciating at times. My work and substance abuse were the only two things I could use to cope with my dark side. My last wakeup call came after having locked myself in my apartment for days drinking and partying, just not wanting to live anymore. I wanted it to just simply end. I woke up three days later to a serious reality check. What if I didn't wake up? What if I actually went through with it?

I was introduced to community theater in the fall of 1994. I started to find a sense of peace and joy as this was something, I was still very passionate about. I immersed myself in my profession while adding theater – it was the perfect mix. Work, performing, directing, and choreographing. The theater was the catalyst for getting me back on a path of self-worth and pride. I achieved so many incredible accomplishments working with wonderful community theater groups. I still go through my own struggles from time to time. I was truly blessed to find the courage to leave that dark, chemically dependent world knowing the outcome if I had continued. It's just a matter of what's your attitude at that moment in your life. I found a sense of peace. Today, I'm with a wonderful man, Joshua. We've been together fourteen years and married seven. We live in Cape Coral, Florida with our kids: Zoie, Zorro, and Zelda.

Every one of us has our own unique journey. Mine certainly was filled with rocking the boat through the years. We deal with challenges and breakthroughs in various ways. Today discussions about mental wellness are becoming more prevalent as many are looking for guidance and there is so much more for those who seek it. This negative stigma is shifting as brave celebrities share their stories. More and more people are coming out looking for help. However, there is still much more work that must be done, and many roads to travel helping spread the good word.

I will forever continue on my mental wellness journey as "mental illness" is still a pandemic that must be destigmatized.

I honestly believe every human being has been impacted by mental illness during their journey. There are so many factors that bring on a multitude of mental illness issues. Everyone's trigger is uniquely different. What I'm now embracing is being able to step back, ask questions, learn, observe and be compassionate about others' situations.

For any male struggling, if you're reading this, rest assured you're not alone it does get better. If you need to talk, reach out. I know for many years I had no one to talk to, I'm here to help provide support.

I'm learning and understanding more about being a Mental Wellness Advocate. Today and moving forward Mental Wellness IS The NEW Physical Health.

Acknowledgments and Dedication

I'd like to acknowledge the following:

Special thanks to Kim Bolton LaMontagne who provided me this golden opportunity.

To my parents, you have been there no matter what, supporting, encouraging and loving from the very beginning. Humbled to be your first-born.

To my brothers, we may not be at each other's sides but always in my heart.

To Dawn, all I can say is unconditionally and AAF.

To Jackie, the sister we never had. It started with WPC, you the catalyst to my well-being journey.

To my extended family and friends who have supported me along the way no matter what.

To my new humanitarian tribe, more chapters on the road to Servant Leader.

And finally Joshua my incredible, amazing, loving husband and best friend ever. I will forever be grateful from the first day you entered my life. You have stuck with me along this amazing journey of LOVE.

About Jeffrey E. Berger

Jeffrey E. Berger. is a humanitarian and an independent wellness partner with Amare Global, the first holistic mental health company that focuses specifically on the microbiome (gut-brain axis). he is humbled to be associated with this mission-based company which strives to create a holistic wellness platform that connects a purpose-driven community of passionate people.

In August 2016, he realized that traveling a traditional path of working in corporate America was not in alignment with his personal growth needs, both mentally and emotionally. His personal achievements, ultimate goals of making a significant difference philanthropically, personally and spiritually were not being met. He is fortunate now to be associated with an incredible community that has as its core values love, integrity, innovation, humility, and service.

There has been such a stigma over the years concerning mental illness; it is a pandemic that needs to be lifted with grace and dignity for those living with this challenge. He has started to educate and guide people through his online, free "Gut-Mind Workshop – The Mental Wellness Revolution" and "Getting to the Root of It" series that addresses the microbiome and its association to mental wellness.

His hope is to help make whatever impact he can by doing his personal best, sharing with those struggling with challenges to their health. We must learn to deal with the negativity associated with mental illness. Knowledge and a positive approach can remove a significant roadblock to mental wellness.

CONTACT INFO:

- https://www.facebook.com/jeffrey.e.berger

- facebook.com/MentalWellnessGladiator

- https://www.linkedin.com/in/jeffreyeberger/

- jeffrey@nulife.biz

- #MentalWellnessGladiator

Xavier Whitford

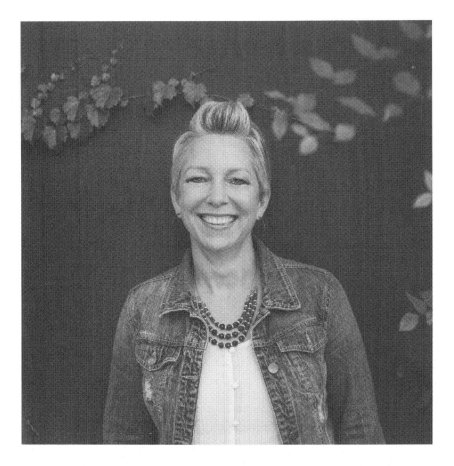

Transforming Wounds into Wisdom

By Xavier Whitford

My life has not been easy and I have experienced enough pain and loss to last a lifetime or so I thought until the day my worst nightmare became reality and I lost my 19-year-old son, Tommy, to suicide. I considered myself a survivor. I survived being raised by an alcoholic mother and without a father. I survived being sexually abused several times as a child. I survived being raped at the age of 14, while I was in a drug treatment facility. I survived teen years of drinking, drugs, and dangerous circumstances. I survived the loss of a husband who died in a drunk driving accident, leaving me a widow to raise our 3-year-old little boy and my daughter, who I was 3 months pregnant with. I thought I was strong and could handle anything that life had to toss at me, until the day I found my beautiful boy dead.

As a toddler Tommy was always smiling and acting silly. Everyone who came in contact with him fell in love with his bright smile and soulful green eyes. However, the traumatic loss of his dad at such a young age affected him greatly. He struggled with anger and sadness over the years and was finally diagnosed with depression and anxiety at 10-years-old.

August 18, 2014 started off like any other day, I woke up, had my coffee, and headed to work. About 11 am, I received a text from my son's girlfriend that they had been in a bad argument and she left.

My son posted he was "worthless" on social media and wasn't answering his phone when I tried to call him. I decided to go check on him. Never at any point had I considered he would not be alive when I arrived. I expected to walk in on him sleeping or listening to music, which is what he often did when he was upset. What I found instead was my son's lifeless body.

The terror of those moments and wounds they created changed the trajectory of my life forever. My mind engraved every moment and imprisoned every detail. As if the pain of seeing my beautiful baby boy cold and blue repeating in my brain was not enough, the vision of my beautiful daughter's face as it registered what had happened to her big brother was on repetition as well. As a mother, our life's mission is to care and protect our children. As if experiencing the reality that my son suffered unimaginable pain that made him believe life wasn't worth living was not sufficient, I also had the reality that my daughter had to survive a major deficit in her life on the first day of her Junior year of High School. Suicide should never be an option. The pain is temporary and yet ending your life is permanent and will forever affect the lives of everyone who knows and loves you. It was excruciating watching her world unravel as news of what her brother had done was blasted across social media in a matter of minutes and no ability to predict or brace her for the impact this was going to have in her life going forward. Relationships she had spent her life building were being shattered due to a cultural lack of understanding suicide. I knew in that moment that things needed to change.

I recognize now that my son could not have known that I would be the one who found him that day or the immense pain it would have initiated. Tommy never would have wanted me or anyone he loved to experience that pain and trauma, but the reality is we did. The many questions and what if scenarios consumed me. I felt like a failure as a mother for not protecting my baby boy from this illness. I felt like I should have known and done more. I believe with all my heart that God recognized that I was resilient enough to handle finding my son that dreadful day and my faith foundation would be a tremendous part of enduring the pain of this enormous loss. In many ways I am thankful it was me and not someone else.

I had always been a person who could control my thoughts and emotions, but this was different. Months after losing Tommy, I found myself consumed with panic, terror, and anxiety to the point I could no longer function. I had no control over what was happening to my mind and body. There were so many instances where I was triggered and it made sense; an ambulance siren, the phone ringing, or certain words and smells. However, there are often things that activate the trauma that you can't anticipate. My family and friends didn't and quite honestly couldn't understand when I tried to explain the tormenting feeling. My husband was my greatest support during this time. Although he didn't understand what I was going through he was always there encouraging me to seek help and reminding me we were going to get through this. Up to this point I had been seeing a grief counselor and going to suicide survivors support group, all of which helped with certain aspects of my grief. However, I realized that wasn't enough. After spending an hour curled up in a ball sobbing and shaking uncontrollably on the bathroom floor at work, I finally embraced the idea of seeing a doctor that specializes in trauma. That doctor diagnosed me with PTSD. I guess it's no surprise that the trauma was more than my brain could process. No mother should have to find their child that way.

Thankfully, the doctor I was connected with was the leading trauma therapist in our area specializing in EMDR. Eye Movement Desensitization and Reprocessing (EMDR) is a psychotherapy treatment that was originally designed to alleviate the distress associated with traumatic memories. During EMDR therapy the individual focuses on emotionally disturbing material in brief sequential doses while simultaneously focusing on an external stimulus. Therapist directed lateral eye movements are the most commonly used external stimulus and what was used on me. I was not convinced it was going to work, but I was willing to try anything to gain some normalcy in my life again. How could holding pulsating buzzers in my hand and thinking about the trauma help at all? Well it did. I noticed improvement right away and with each visit the flashbacks became less encompassing. The most interesting part of EMDR for me was the connection of trauma to our body. I learned after the first treatment that physical pain accompanies the mental healing process. I held my pain in my right shoulder because it was directly connected to the trauma. You see the day I found my son hanging, I held him up on my right shoulder while I called 911. It felt like I held my son's lifeless body for hours, but I was later told it was only a few minutes. This form of therapy is not right for everyone, but I believe EMDR was right for me and saved my life. I still remember every detail of every moment of that day and the grief that accompanies that loss, but it no longer devours me.

I have found that this personal experience with PTSD has provided me an avenue to better understand individuals living with mental illness and the lack of control they have. Much like a heart attack, you might feel it coming but you cannot stop it from happening. All you can do is learn from the process and do what you can to treat the symptoms in hopes you can prevent it from happening again.

I was somewhat familiar with what Tommy's needs were from losing his Dad, or so I thought. I was doing everything I'd been told to do by his doctors and believed his depression was under control with the new medication he had been prescribed. I didn't know much about mental illness or suicide and it was never on my scope for educational knowledge beyond what Tommy's doctors were advising in relation to his depression. However, as my family and I were thrown into a world where one is forced to try to comprehend the incomprehensible, and deal with the after effects of the trauma, education and knowledge helped. I struggled to figure out all the "whys" from a life that was so full of love but remained one he didn't find worth living.

Most of what I have learned has been from listening to individuals who fight mental illness every day. They have helped me understand in greater detail the lies that our brains tell us when we are battling with feelings of worthlessness and hopelessness. I have learned the signs and symptoms of depression and the risk factors that lead to suicide. Many of these things I brushed off as just a teenage phase with Tommy, but now I know differently. Never in all the years my son was in and out of counselors, doctors, and rehabs did anyone tell me that depression is the number one leading cause of suicide. Now I know. This is why I find it so important to shatter the silence, end the stigma, and educate individuals so they don't have to suffer the same fate as we did.

So, what did I do with this experience and knowledge? I've learned to use my fear and pain as a catapult to take action and ignite change. In the days and months after losing my son I literally had to remind myself to breathe. I felt controlled and suffocated by the fear that consumed me, but after finding the right treatment to help me work through the trauma, I was able to transform the wounds I experienced into wisdom to help others. Instead of allowing the fear to control me, to paralyze me, I used its energy to take action and fight to make a difference.

I found out very quickly that the stigma that surrounds mental illness and suicide is ever present and prevents individuals from feeling comfortable in reaching out for help. I promptly recognized that silence is the biggest obstacle to overcome the stigma so people feel at ease asking for help. If we break the silence that surrounds these topics, it opens up a dialogue that will allow individuals to feel more comfortable in talking about what they are experiencing. Talking about my personal story of great loss, PTSD, and pain puts me in a very vulnerable position. Helping others by creating support groups puts me in a sensitive spot. Speaking in front of hundreds of individuals on the factors that lead to suicide is not at all what I envisioned doing in my life. But all of that is not worse than sitting back and doing nothing. The amazing thing is that this shift in feeling, this shift in thinking, isn't really about confidence in my ability to survive anything. It isn't really about trying to tell myself never to be afraid. It's not about remaining calm and peaceful. Sometimes, fear is actually healthy. It's about taking the fear and turning it into something powerful. It's about not allowing the fear to control you and being willing to ask and seek help when you need it. It's about learning to be your biggest advocate. Sometimes our deepest pain can create our greatest purpose.

While I had support from friends and family, my greatest source of guidance was found in my faith. I don't understand why I had to lose my son to suicide, however, from the very moment I realized Tommy was gone I felt in my heart that God was going to use this for His glory. And He has. God called me to be strong enough to speak out about this tragedy, to bring light into the darkness, and allow Him to utilize me for a greater purpose than I could imagine.

I have come to realize that I need to ask myself an important question when paralyzed by fear; "What if you do nothing? What if your action helps to save a life? What if you are the answer to the problem?" Using these powerful questions not only sheds some light on whether or not my fears are reality, but also helps put in perspective the fact that doing nothing can cause more harm than good. This is also the case when we find ourselves struggling with grief, depression, substance use, anxiety, PTSD, or any other mental battle. We have to be willing to share our story and ask for help when we are not ok. Staying stuck, paralyzed by fear and pain, is no longer an option. Believing that it will get better on its own and not wanting to be a burden to others is no longer an option. We have to make a choice to transform our fear into action and be willing to fight.

Our wounds provide a story that can be used to help others and ourselves. It seems strange to be thankful for the wounds I have experienced in my life, but I am, because each wound has taught me something important. I am not the same person I was and never will be, but each experience I have been through has got me to where I am today. I have become a person who can relate and understand others who are fighting a mental battle. I have become a person who has deep compassion and empathy for others who are often isolated and stereotyped. I have become a person who doesn't just survive but thrive in many aspects of my life. I have learned that each and every moment matters and every life matters. No one is meant to walk this journey alone and no one has to.

It doesn't matter who you are, life will leave battle wounds. If you are reading this and you feel like you have so many scars and wounds that there is no way you will ever fully heal, I am here to say you can and will! You are not alone and the truth is wounds come with living this life. It's what we do with those wounds that defines who we are and our future. Make a choice to transform your wounds into wisdom and never be afraid to ask for help. It's ok to reach out for help. It's ok to not be ok. What's not ok is trying to face those battles alone. With every battle it takes an army of soldiers to win. Build your defense by reaching out to those around you that can inspire, encourage, and support you when you need it. Be your biggest advocate and never be afraid to ask for help. No one walks away from a battle without wounds, but those wounds can be used for wisdom and become a powerful tool for survival.

Acknowledgements and Dedication

I would like to extend my heartfelt gratitude to my husband and daughter for always supporting me in following my heart to share our journey in hopes to inspire and encourage others. A special thanks to Crystal, Anne, and Tonya for continuously urging me to write. Thanks to my amazing friends and family who've supported and encouraged me on my mission to break the stigma and end the silence around mental illness and suicide.

I am incredibly grateful for all those who have shared their personal stories to help educate me along the way. I am eternally grateful for the love and mercy of Jesus Christ and the purpose He has instilled in me through the pain. Everything I do is to honor God and my precious boy, Tommy, who I miss dearly every single minute. I love you Tommy and hope I've made you proud.

About Xavier Whitford

Xavier (pronounced Sha vee air) Whitford has spent the past five years devoting her life to helping others who live with mental illness. Sharing her insights and personal story of losing her son, Tommy, to suicide as well as her own journey through depression, anxiety, and PTSD as a result of that great loss. Xavier has taken her pain and turned it into a purpose to cultivate a deeper understanding of the nature of living with mental illness and suicidal thoughts.

Xavier is a wife of a Pastor, mother of two, and Gigi to a beautiful little princess. She has spoken at many schools, churches and organizations inspiring and educating groups of all ages to end the stigma surrounding mental illness and on the factors that lead to suicide. Xavier helps arm individuals within communities with support and training. Her personal story, tireless commitment, and passion to improve support and education around these topics has made her a powerful advocate to the mental health community.

Xavier is a teacher, advocate, and a board member with the National Alliance on Mental Illness, Northern Illinois Chapter. As a Mental Health First Aid Instructor, Xavier teaches members of the public how to help a person developing a mental health problem, experiencing a worsening of an existing mental health problem or in a mental health crisis. In her role as a facilitator for Teen Mental Health Groups and Grief Support Groups, she provides an opportunity to talk with, and listen to, others who know the personal nature of living with mental illness and grief in a safe and non-judgmental environment. Xavier is a writer, blogger, and suicide loss survivor.

Kathy Clark

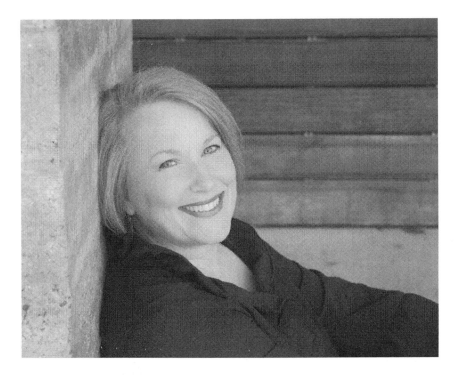

Self-Debting

By Kathy Clark

Something innate within me from a very early age began the habit of being so self-aware that I began moving the puzzle pieces within me to maneuver and manipulate the puzzle pieces externally to the point that I had displaced every puzzle piece that mattered to me. Essentially, you mattered more to me than I mattered to me. This is so important to begin to understand that my "being ok" was so compromised that it became a chronic condition and prevalent in the majority of my thoughts from a very early age. Why does this matter for what follows? Because, it compromised the very nature of situations and events that caused depression, anxiety, a sense of not belonging, or being in the "gap, with feeling isolated and thoughts that were not self-loving or compassionate.

I think a lot of my suffering over the years might have been stopped sooner had I known that "not being ok" was acceptable, normal, and a part of life. I find that society, in general, promotes not to be so down and to "lighten up". If you're an empath like me, where absorbing the emotions and moods of others is first nature, it can even make "lightening up" even more challenging because I could not define the line on where you ended and I began.

Living in the crevice of life is quite isolating and separating. I saw life buzzing by, happy and joyous while I felt the energy of all of the positivity and excitement while in the crevice. Seeing people get married, having precious children, laughing, and enjoying life. While I was observing it all, I desperately wanted all of that. I kept marching forward hoping that one day it would stick. Sure, I had moments of achievement of graduating nursing school, which was probably one of the happiest days of my life. Somehow, I would slip back into not being ok and not having the feeling of belonging as Brene' Brown speaks of.

I've been told that I'm intelligent, funny, pretty, compassionate, and many other things as well. And for some reason I hear those things and am flattered. And yet, I do not integrate them into the core of me. Like those traits are sticky notes that are put on me. I see them and feel them on me but they are ever-so-gently adhered to me easy to be removed by the next wave negative thoughts and opinions of others. Sometimes they were drowning sounds like locusts in the hot summer days. I wish I had a penny for every time I heard, "you have a lot going for you, why aren't you happy" or "you keep looking back and dwelling on the past". Like for me, was that even an option for me not to do those things? The responsibility I felt for others' wellbeing and happiness was so innate that this is where the belonging went off the tracks. How could I belong when I poured every ounce of me outward. And, how…how do I stop doing for others and put me first? What a proposition that was and I was completely terrified to put me first. This is probably the most mind-boggling thing. Why am I so afraid of being me, knowing me, and being ok with me? It's time that I begin to explore the why of those questions.

I was once told, "you love people and you don't know why you need them." When people told me that they loved me, I often wondered what I had done to earn that love. Somehow I began to see a huge disconnect in my ability to allow people into my inner circle. I began putting the pieces of the puzzle together that I was so terrified of abandonment that at an early age I began disassociating and being of service to others. One thing I can tell you for certain is that I feel everything very deeply and I always have. As a child, I could not kill even the smallest bug that would cross my path. I was one of those very sensitive types. Seeing hurt and anguish in the world also hurt me from a deep visceral place. I began to wall up those emotions because I did not feel safe having those feelings. If you envision a castle, my heart and emotions were behind curtains of stone where a bridge allowed a very small opening for just a small amount of light to enter and surrounded by water to prevent any attacks on the very tender heart that was guarded. Beyond the moat, which everyone was telling me, were fields of grass that were very lush and the color of emeralds. There were also beautiful gardens that were tended to by the townspeople. In order for connection to occur, I had to trust that my heart which felt so battered and bruised after handing it to others to care for would be ok. What I really didn't trust is that I could learn to love and take care of me in a way that would allow someone in and I realized that the price to pay for walling off my heart which was actually killing me. It killed my spirit, joy, creativity and eventually my soul. Remember the scene in Alita: Battle Angel where she was offering her heart that could power the city to the very person who had a bounty on her heart? That was me.

To drown out the hurt, I had to find something to replace the hurt with feeling better. The first relief I had in a chemical was food. I seemed to obsess about where my next meal would come from and then would begin to think that the quantity of food was not going to be enough. Looking back now, I see that it was a protection that I could obtain some level of security through food so I began serving lunch in school to ensure that I would have lunch. Then, the real magic entered into my life…alcohol. It seemed to magically change me immediately upon the first drink. Once alcohol hit my blood stream, it was like a switch had been flipped on and liquid happiness would course through my veins. At that moment, I forgot all of the worries and the obsessive thoughts seemed to quiet. Between the ages of 21 and 35 I lived a life of daily drinking. The torture of Sméagol and Gollum battling for my attention was torture on a daily basis when I didn't drink. By the time I was close to 35, I began seeing chemical dependency signs and I was about done with the elixir that was killing me. I wound up putting it down and then the feelings I worked so hard on killing had resurfaced with a vengeance. And, they had to. Somehow, making this decision deep within allowed all of the miracles to begin pouring down from heaven.

I heard Marianne Williams say in a podcast…that when you hold on to something so tightly, you are not allowing God to replace it with what He wants for you. The moment you put the 'thing' down that is keeping you from the sunlight of the spirit, He can begin to shower you with those gifts which are far better than you can ever imagine. That began to happen. One day at a time just saying no to something I thought was my best friend. Fast forward my life at the 11-year mark somehow opened up my inner shine that came with doing the next right thing day-after-day between 2002 and 2013. I couldn't see it or feel it. I relied on others telling me that I was different and that I was glowing. I was in nursing school, riding motorcycles, and surrounded by people I loved and I began to know what being loved 'felt' like and it was intoxicating. I am not going to say that I was never loved prior to this time, but this was the first time I knew what it felt like to openly love and then also receive love and be vulnerable. For one year, I beamed happiness like never before.

The year 2014 would have been the pinnacle of that happiness and it came crashing down in a matter of three months. And, what I didn't realize at the time was that He was pruning every branch that was not producing fruit. The relationship I was in and had really loved being in saw me walking away because we were not compatible. I moved out without much of my possessions because I gave them up and failed nursing school. I walked away from motorcycles because I had two herniated discs in my neck which was so painful that riding was not an option. Nearly everything that I thought was important to me was pruned. This was so painful. I learned at this crucial juncture of my life that women were the most powerful healers even if it meant just sitting in their presence. I cried and cried. I walked in grocery stores with tears streaming down my face. God made it very clear that this was one of those times that He needed me very close to Him to heal those places that were so deeply hidden in the castle so we could expose it to the sunlight to grow. There were parts of me that I questioned...was this a part of me or something that I mirrored from someone else to gain acceptance and love? So, the next brave thing to do was to remove these labels to sit with me. This time the crevice became the valley. For eight months, I cried and sat in the valley. This was the first time that I truly learned that it was ok not to be ok. That not being ok meant that I was healing and feeling through everything the alcohol drowned. Little did I know that this pruning period happens to so many over the course of life. No one is immune. I didn't realize as well that it was preparation for another time in my life that I was quickly coming upon.

I faced another challenge that I was very unprepared for. I began a depression in 2017 that quickly worsened in 2018. Being in the medical arena, I knew the steps to take. I did everything conventional and non-conventional to relieve the symptoms of wicked lethargy, depression, suicidal thoughts, and no desire to do anything I had enjoyed previously. I tried SSRI's and I had side effects to those which I never had before. I tried ADD medication because my thoughts were like popcorn kernels in a frying pan. Any stone that I saw, I turned it over to see if that was the solution. The amount of rocks that I overturned could probably fill up an aquarium. Then, one suggestion was made to me by a nursing instructor. She provided me the name of a healthcare provider that dealt with hormones and wellness. I could barely stay awake in my appointment and then she read through the report, she said she was going to treat me for hypothyroidism. For three months, I kept pushing forward and taking the medications and then one day the clouds disappeared. I called my friend, Kim LaMontagne on Thanksgiving Day and let her know it was over. Such as the ending scene in Labyrinth where Sarah looks at David Bowie's character, Jareth, and says "You have no power over me." She is then quickly transitioned back to her lovely life dancing with all of her friends. That was the realization that I had where chemical imbalances wreaked havoc over my life. It impaired my ability to experience joy and even perform simple tasks. Even to this day, if I miss a dose of my thyroid medication, I begin to have great anxiety because I refuse to go there again. I was ready to jump in and experience life again.

With that one call to Kim, I was invited to participate in my first contributing author experience, had finished up my coaching certification and had a new lease on life. Just as I was about to enjoy life again, I was faced with a job loss. Once again, a pruning. At this point, I think it's a blessing and the experience is maybe for another book when I'm ready. But this time, I'm moving forward with doing the next right thing in a different capacity. I gain strength, yet again. I'm beginning to understand that the pruning precedes rapid growth and maturity. Some of you may be thinking…sheesh, she must have ninja level wisdom and I'm sure the answer to that is, "hold my root beer, watch this" as God puts me in another season of growth.

What I want to encourage you to know, my dear, is that everyone you see in life goes through many prunings in their lives. It feels like the worst thing that can happen to you and the only reason why is there "is" a death that is occurring. It's a death of what is not serving you. It provides an avenue of healing and openness for God to give you what will serve you and others. It's a time for self-reflection and nurturing like you've never experienced before. This was the hardest part for me, to put me first. Heck, no one can do that for you on a continuous basis and I had to realize that to even expect that was pure selfishness. I didn't come for this journey to throw up the white flag and give up. Even though I did it many times, I would get sick of myself if I didn't try again. Adventure is my middle name and, oh yes, I've also been called brave and tenacious…heck, I'm not giving up those because I'm tired.

What is it you want out of life? Where did you give up and abandon those very sweet dreams you once had? Our only hope is that you do what makes you happy and let the authenticity shine outward. There is no fitting in ever…EVER. You fit in where you choose to be. If they don't like it then they are threatened by your authenticity and jealous because their own walls are preventing them from truly living life. Group think is stink think. Just don't go there. This is where I'm becoming ok with me. Yes, I'm an empath, I love hard and deep and I will get hurt over and over again because there are disappointments in life. Living safe made me drunk…on a daily basis and not in a good way. Let the adrenaline flow…let is flow through you readily and do what excites you. Don't stop doing what made you laugh at the age of three, five or even 13. So, dear, tell me…what makes you happy? I want to know.

Acknowledgments

I've had so many wonderful people in my life to support and love me during the times I was not ok. These people will forever be in my heart and I have an immense amount of gratitude for their ability to just hold presence to let me be me in any state. Without each of you, I would not be where I am today. Many blessings to you and your family.

About Kathy Clark

Kathy Clark, BSN, RN, is a speaker, scholar, writer, executive, and passionate community volunteer. Kathy is a member of the American Nurses Association, National Alliance on Mental Illness and hones her skills as a Registered Nurse by traveling to third world countries to work with medical aid mission teams. Presently, her thirst for knowledge is quenched by her studies toward a Master of Science with a concentration in Executive Coaching, and by her intentional openness to finding wisdom in the everyday. A self-described empath and extrovert, Kathy has learned to make room for serendipity by listening to the small voice, the intuition that tells her to strike up a conversation with an unlikely stranger. In these encounters the ordinary becomes extraordinary and her circuitous path to professional, personal and scholarly fulfillment is enriched.

With her coaching certification through the International Coaching Federation, Kathy has eagerly begun her endeavor of personal and professional development with her brand Kathy Clark RN, www.kathyclarkrn.com, and programs through IBA Coaching, www.ibacoaching.com, Imagine Believe Achieve.

You can also find her on Facebook, LinkedIn, Instagram, and Pinterest at Kathy Clark RN, or kathy@kathyclarkrn.com.

A native of New Orleans, Kathy currently resides in the Houston area where animal lovers know her through her volunteer efforts, rescuing and fostering abandoned animals and housing as many as six, four-legged dependents at once.

Denise L. Curan

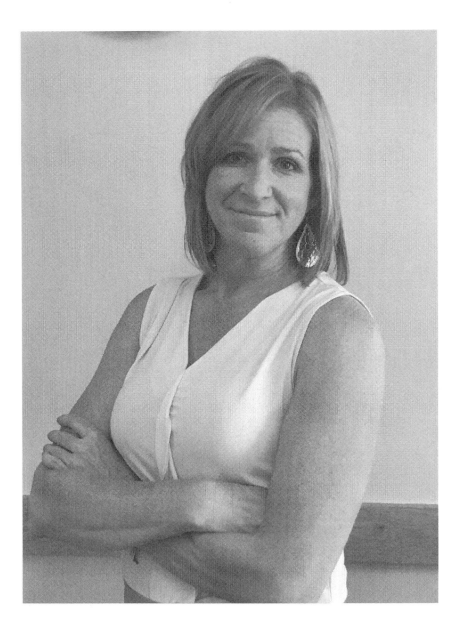

I Am Not Collateral Damage

By Denise L. Curan

The grinding of the metal lulled me as I slowly rocked us back and forth on the expansive redwood swing set. This had been a gift to the kids the previous Christmas from Santa. We had never known how to do things small when it came to them. Most of this was due to the devastatingly poor way that I had been brought up. When having access to basic necessities put me at odds with all of my peers throughout my childhood, assuring my own children had more than enough was the only way that I wanted them to be able to live.

I reflected on my upbringing and how it had brought me to this point. The intense desire for acceptance and unconditional love. How I had been shown what working hard looked like, but never what happiness felt like. Taught of a God that will help you suffer through the pain, but that pain was inevitable.

The sun was settling in for the evening and our slow-moving reflections were distorted on the patio as we moved gently in time with the rest of the world. I noticed the warm, musty smell that indicated autumn was about to kiss summer. It smelled of dirt and crunchy leaves that crackle when you walk. My breathing was slow and even as I worked to quiet the emotions that I wanted no part of.

I looked at the little hand in mine. The tiny perfect little fingernails, the smooth soft skin in comparison with my own skin that had lines starting to reflect my age. No one would want a hand like that to hold except these babies who knew no better.

Those chubby baby fingers reached up and touched my cheek, wiping away the silent tears that ran down them. Neither of my babies, my daughter was four and my son was two, asked why their Momma cried quietly. They just sat and held on with their innocence as we listened to their Daddy yell inside the house about how terrible I was and how I had ruined his life by being such a loser. On this occasion, I think it might have had something to do with the house not being clean enough.

These were not new words, but the feelings that they created as my children witnessed the emotional abuse that I endured, were overwhelming. I thought that I could save him. I believed that, as his wife, it was sickness and health, even mental health. This is the first moment that I came to believe that the world had no hope. There was only evil. I wished that I had never brought these beautiful little souls into this world.

An idea began to spark, a terrible, horrible thought. They did not have to suffer through this hopeless world and neither did I. All the things that I had worked so hard to overcome from my youth and all of the desires for my future, every prayer that I prayed so diligently, had meant nothing.

In my mind, I thought about taking us all down to the garage and putting us in the car. I would turn their little movie on and start the car. Then I could just wait...........

The only thing that stopped me from acting on this idea, was as the thought of what might happen if someone found us and the little bodies of my children and succumbed to the fumes, but mine had not. There is not a breath that I could take on this earth without them.

I dried my eyes. My heart raged at God for leaving me here after all of my begging to make it better. Then the internal conversation about getting my shit together and stop being the loser that my husband knew I was kicked in. My armor returned. My heart got just a bit harder. This is what surviving looks like.

This was the first time that I had contemplated taking my life, but not the last. It was the only time that I contemplated taking my children's.

This is the collateral damage of what mental illness can do. This is the first time that I have told this story.

Now, as I walk you through these moments, understand that I am only telling my story. The man I had loved enough to create that life with and bring these children into the world with, suffered greatly with his own demons and his story is his to share. His perception of things and understanding of the wounds that were created, are very different from mine.

Now, so many years later, we have both grown and healed in many ways and the person he is today is not the same. It does not change the devastation that his struggles put me through during our marriage.

I had just turned 19 and he had just turned 20 when we met. We grew up together and my soul purpose was to create a happy husband and a happy home for our children. I went so far as to sacrifice my own mental health to try and accomplish this.

Even after this incident with my babies on the swing, it would be almost two years before I told another person what was happening to me. Some had ideas about it, but no one really knew and I did not speak of what went on in my home. I believed I was protecting my family as much as myself from shame and embarrassment. I did not want anyone to know we were not perfect. It would still be another six years later before God would finally give me the strength to end the marriage.

Now if you are reading this, and you have had a single thought of "she should have done.......", you do not deserve to read my story. You have not suffered greatly enough to understand the devastation that can occur in a soul to take you to your darkest places, and unfortunately, you are the reason that I feared so greatly to reach out to someone else until it was almost too late to save myself.

For any of you that feel tears forming in your eye, the lump fill your throat, and the tightness across your chest. This is for you. You are not alone.

I want to go back to that girl on the swing and hold her. I want to tell her that she is loved and that she will survive. I want her to know that there is beauty even in her pain. Since I cannot tell her, I want to tell each of you that have found your way to my story, you are not alone. There is hope even when you cannot see it in the darkness. Your pain will not make sense, but in it you are becoming something more.

My separation was every bit as traumatic and fear inducing as I had anticipated. We all survived. We all walked through the fire stronger and better, my ex-husband included. I would not have made it through without starting to reach out to those around me. I lost many relationships with people that had no idea what truth I had been living. I also learned who I could count on and who truly loved me. I wish I had reached out so much sooner.

I am still in the process of healing. It has been seven years since my marriage has ended and I have to constantly evaluate my thought processes as I navigate new relationships. I have had to learn to love myself and change my internal dialogue to one of love and gentleness. God and I have had to work together to heal that bond, as I felt so alone and unheard for so many years.

The suffering did not end in one step. Selling our home and downsizing to a duplex was shortly followed by the elimination of my position with a company that I had been with for 12 years that had provided a sense of financial security. Each of these hits left me feeling like I continued to swirl in some dark storm.

I began to find spiritual and mental healing through nutrition and physical exercise. The more that I focused in on my physical well being, I noticed my mood improving and my feeling of hope and possibility returning.

People often ask how I can workout at 5am every morning or how I can invest so much commitment to my physical health, the answer is that I do not have a choice. This is my place, my meditation, and my peace. This is the thing that has saved me when nothing else could bring me back. I talk to God on my runs, I push my boundaries at CrossFit, and increasing my physical strength, diminishes so many years of feeling weak and small.

My redemption has been found through caring for my physical self and its ability to spread into so many other areas of self care, such as setting safe boundaries for emotions and the strong female friendships that I have established.

That girl on that swing that wanted to end the pain for her and her babies no longer exists. The strong and capable woman that I am now, wants to find every girl that is hurting and give her hope.

Acknowledgements and Dedication

First and foremost, all of my thanks must go to God for assuring that I am still here today to share my story. Then I must acknowledge by three beautiful children, Lauren, Christian, and Lily, through each of them and their individual light I have learned more about love than I knew possible.

About Denise L. Curran

Denise Curran is the creator of StrongMommyInc. This organization has been created to support the spiritual and mental growth of women and mothers through the use of nutrition and exercise.

Denise believes that physical activity and nutrition play a key factor in the overall satisfaction and capability for emotional and spiritual growth.

Denise has utilized her personal experiences related to struggles and success with utilizing proper diet and exercise as a catalyst for spiritual and mental health to develop a plan to support other women in the same capacity.

Denise is a Registered Nurse with a Master's Degree in Business Administration. She has been actively involved in the use of nutrition and physical exercise in the healing process spanning the critical care environment, long-term care with seniors, the disabled, and all ages in the outpatient and in-home care setting. She has gained this knowledge in the capacity of both the clinician as well as during her Administrative roles.

She has been published in The Journal of Alzheimer's and Other Dementias. Has been an active board member for a Long-term Acute Care Hospital. Currently holds a seat on the Ethics Committee with a Level I Trauma Center and consults annually with two separate teaching institutions regarding their nursing programs and potential for holistic healing.

Frankie Samah

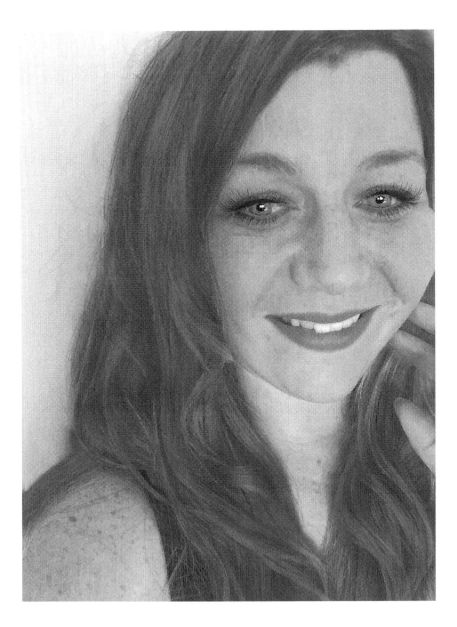

Journey to Happiness

By Frankie Samah

I have a bright orange VW camper van, which we love to spend the summers travelling in. We had travelled to the Outer Hebrides and were blown away with the breath-taking beauty of the Isles. The skies were so big and darkness only came for a short few hours. During the daylight, the heather was blooming on the moorlands that cover the interior of the isles. There is evidence of peat farming everywhere, and around every bend we took, there was a new breath-taking view.

It's in moments like this that I feel so unbelievably blessed with life and the beauty of it. But despite this undeniable beauty of my surroundings, the inability to sleep had travelled with me too.

On one night in particular, I couldn't stop this feeling that someone was coming to push the van over the cliff. I couldn't sleep the whole night, just thinking I had to protect my daughter. When I woke up in the morning and began to process the dream, I realised there were a few reasons why this was completely irrational. Firstly, it's a vehicle that weighs a ton and secondly, we were nowhere near a cliff.

It was here I thought to myself, I have two options- I could either continue to let the past chase me or I need to learn how to come to terms with the past and stop it from manifesting itself in other ways.

It's here I decided to go on my journey of self-love and self-acceptance.

Over the past years, I had been putting on a brave face. I was a single mum and I worried about everything. I worried about buying a house, career trajectories, finding someone to fall in love with, being financially solvent and presenting to the world that we were doing just fine. As time went by my brain couldn't continue with that level of intensity. I began to not think of where I needed to be or where other people thought I should be. These were insignificant to the need to stay alive. I began to debate my existence until the suicide ideation took over my entire thought process. I could barely leave the house and I wanted to be a shut-in. I tried to close the door to the world.

I decided to try and increase my career prospects and went back to university as a mature student. After a few months of returning to university, while I was driving, a lorry drove into the back of my car. Although physically, everything healed and was ok, psychologically it intensified my anxiety. As a result of this, the insurance company sent me for a psychological examination.

After multiple questions, the psychologist diagnosed me with post-traumatic stress disorder from multiple traumas and severe anxiety.

It had been ten years since I walked out on my abusive husband. That incident that forced me into action was when my daughter was only 15 months old. I was walking around the living room, bouncing her in my arms to try to get her to sleep. We had a glass panelled door in the living room that separated it from the hall. My husband came up behind me and grabbed my head into the glass, while our daughter was still in my arms. Glass covered us. I was utterly taken aback by shock. After this, I went to stay with friends and eventually, a women's refuge. I continued to go to work, and my daughter to nursery as if everything was still ok. On the inside, I was breaking.

All through our lives, we are taught once you've had a good education, you will find a good job, then you will be able to buy the right home, and then you will be happy. We are so deeply conditioned to what we should do from an early age, but this is just collective thoughts from society — the ideal fairy tale ending.

This aspiration for the picture-perfect life doesn't prepare you for when things go sideways. It doesn't tell you that this 'happiness goal' is a mirage in the desert. You can keep pedalling for it faster and faster, but as soon as you think it's attainable, it starts to evaporate.

It didn't help that others had opinions about what was going on in my life. It's only now with reflection I can look back at their opinions and see it was ridiculous. People were projecting their feelings and fears on to me. To be made to feel like I wouldn't ever be properly happy unless I was back on the track of 'life' and seeking the same things is complete nonsense.

It's only now that I see a huge part of happiness comes from being utterly free of the expectations of other people, and to a much deeper extent, of myself.

My friend lost her sister in a tragic car accident, and after it happened, friends became upset with her grieving process. I remember our mutual friend telling her it's been two years now, and you should be over it now. As if grief had a time limit. In society, there is a lack of compassion and misunderstanding of mental health that people are pushed to mask how they are feeling and shamed into not showing their real emotions. The more we wear this mask, the more dissonance it creates.

We do not need to process our emotions quicker; there isn't a life scale that has a tick box. Our existence may be rooted in hormones and chemicals, but we certainly cannot live our lives by following mathematical formula.

Over the next ten years, I continued pretending everything was ok. Society tells us to compartmentalise or medicate our life, troubles, our sadness. But no matter how good I was at putting it in the metaphorical box and moving on- the underlying trauma was still there. It manifested itself in other ways such as severe anxiety, panic attacks and extreme self-loathing.

I had created this scenario to protect my ego from more harm and judgements. I had told myself that everyone around me had chosen traditional life choices. Therefore, they were not equipped to question my life choices. So, to live the life I had wanted, I had to remove myself from other people, then I would be free from their judgements. I would surround myself with silence and isolation.

With hindsight, I can see that there is a clear distinction between making an active choice to live a life of solitude versus a choice to live alone because you are afraid of people. One is empowering, and the other…well… it's sad.

For so long, I was mad at my ex-husband for letting us down. I was upset this perfect life I had dreamt of had been taken away from me. I am angry he has never been punished. But I was mostly mad at myself for letting someone treat me like that, for taking advantage of me, for using me. I hated myself the most.

Having the self-hate dialogue wasn't useful to me- I had to take control of my own narrative.

I no longer wanted to live a life full of apathy or regret. Even though I still had the tidal pressures of life around me, there was a new-found beauty in the fragility of living that I had seemed to have taken for granted.

One of the tools I found to help me process my emotions was writing. Writing had never been in my life's plan. While I had returned to the university as a mature student, a professor gave me advice to set up a Tumblr account anonymously and write freely. I found myself free from judgement. In the same way, reading books is a conduit into a million new worlds. Writing helped me articulate how I related to this world. It allowed me to unfold my fragility in a world where I felt muted and amplify my voice to remind myself I am who I am.

I told my story. I had been bullied for being sensitive, too fat, too ugly, too kind, too vulnerable. I had built up walls to protect myself. I thought I am not worthy of being welcomed into their life. I was not worthy of being loved. I wrote about my pain. As hard as it was, it healed me. The deeper I went, the higher my courage rose. I was turning pain into something beautiful.

This gave me conviction. Our world needs more people who are not afraid to be human. People who aren't afraid to be vulnerable and stand in front of the world and say, this is who I am, raise their voice and say this is what happened to me and this is how I overcame it.

And one of the biggest things, I am doing by writing this is saying to the person who oppressed me and to everyone who witnessed his oppression that this should never have happened to me. I did not deserve that. I am telling everyone who is reading this, anything that happens to you that's not ok, is not ok. Regardless of who says you deserved it, or it was your fault it happened, or I don't know whether to believe you or not. You lived your story, just as I have lived mine. No one has the right to take away my story from me, as when you take that away, you take away that person I am becoming. And I love the person I am becoming.

For so long after the trauma of the abuse, people would tell me, I want the old Frankie back. I thought if I changed how I dressed, how I talked, or how I acted, I would find a place that I would fit back in. That by conforming to society norms, I'd find a community or at least try to find that old Frankie. Writing allowed me to permit myself to be creative and to be un-shamefully myself- my anxiety about making the 'right choices' lessened. I couldn't spend my life trying to meet some outdated standards. Stepping out of these chains we have created for ourselves is terrifying but incredibly liberating.

Our brains have one goal- to keep us safe and alive. Our subconscious mind works to make this happen. The neural firings in the brain cause us to repeat the same thoughts, experience the same emotions, and then we repeat that behaviour. It's the part of our subconscious mind called the homeostatic impulse. Homeostasis is our body's way of staying balanced. The homeostatic impulse controls things we do without thinking, such as our body temperature, breathing and heart rate. It also works mentally, keeping us thinking and behaving in a way that is consistent with our past.

This is why so many people feel stuck- they are. This is why the journey of self-love is so difficult. When we start to end an old habit, such as self-loathing, in the beginning, we may experience some mental resistance, then the mental chatter begins. We convince ourselves we need that habit or it's not that bad, or I deserve that self-loathing because I am a terrible person. The first week feels stressful, and mental resistance becomes endless. But we need to practice separation from our thoughts, or we will operate as most people do, that thoughts are a reality. We allow our mind to control our behaviour and deem that being without that habit is too stressful. The path to healing is to push past these thoughts, rather than identify with them. This means small steps in our own time, with daily acts to break up patterning regardless of how triggering this will be in the beginning. As new neural pathways are formed, the resistance fades.

We have in this society an ingrained belief of love being comfortable and effortless, which for some people it is. But love isn't one-dimensional. Love is a state of being and operates on each end of the spectrum; from anger to perfect happiness. There are always going to be parts of us that are easier to love than other parts. Maybe it's how ridiculously funny you are or how you can always see the kindness in people. But real self-love is being fully conscious and aware of the darker parts of our personality. The parts of ourselves none of us like to admit are in us. These are the parts that can lead us to self-destruct when things get tough. Behaviour is often not binary, like good or bad, or the angel and the demon on our shoulders like Freud made us believe. It's usually the insidious stuff that presses down on our life, that causes us to act out in specific ways, like drinking too much or the inability to respect our boundaries. Our darker selves can be a master of covering itself. Self-love comes from accepting what we are doing is terrible for us, but it's me, and I need to find out what it is, so I can stop making the same mistakes.

If a lesson keeps presenting itself to you, again and again, you must allow yourself to experience it truly. Be present and breathe through it and look for what it is trying to teach you. Push through the emotions and invite that growth from within. Through that experience, we will identify and confront the barriers that keep us from love, peace and happiness. This is growth; this is how we learn to heal, how we learn to love ourselves. This is the act of becoming.

I have now found someone I want to share my life with. I love him not because society tells me I have to be in love, or I am only a worthy human if someone loves me. I love him because of his qualities. He is kind, and he is loyal. There is a saying that when you have met your 'soul mate' you have met your half, but this implies that we are only a 'whole' human when we are in a relationship. I refute this idea because as I have come on my journey, I have realised I don't need him to be in my life to be happy, but I want him there. I don't have to be alone, and self-love also comes from interacting with people who know you. Not just the surface level you, but the person deep underneath. Our relationship is not built on need, but on giving each other the freedom for personal growth and creativity. Our love is built on memories and laughter. It might not be the conventional love that was written in storybooks, but it is our story.

When you actually live something, you can't return to who you were before you lived it. Healing is a lifelong journey. We can choose to go past the conditioning, the emotional addictions and the ego to create a version of self in line with who we actually are. A past version of myself would not recognise me now. I've shredded the avatar of myself and met my authentic self.

Acknowledgements

I want to thank my beautiful Ameera, you are my dream come true.

To my beautiful partner, with your love and support I continue to heal, grow and evolve.

I want to think my Mum, Dad, and especially my big sister for your endless love.

To my Kaylie I would not of been here without you.

To Deniyal for always helping me believe in myself.

I can not thank you enough for what you have all done for me.

About Frankie Samah

Frankie Samah is a children's book author, she owns a tapas bar with her big sister. She is a psychology teacher and takes a keen interest in researching psychological interventions for mental health. She regularly contributes to different psychology magazines.

Frankie lives in Mid-Wales, with her daughter, her two puppies and her bright orange camper van, Reggie.

As an advocate for mental health awareness, Frankie aspires to use positive psychology and encourage others to never give up on themselves. We can all be whatever we want to be- all we have to do is believe in ourselves.

Follow Frankie on Instagram, Twitter and on her blog. Her handles are below-

Blog: www.frankiesamah.com

Instagram: @frankiesamah

Twitter: @frankiesamah

Sarah Blackburn

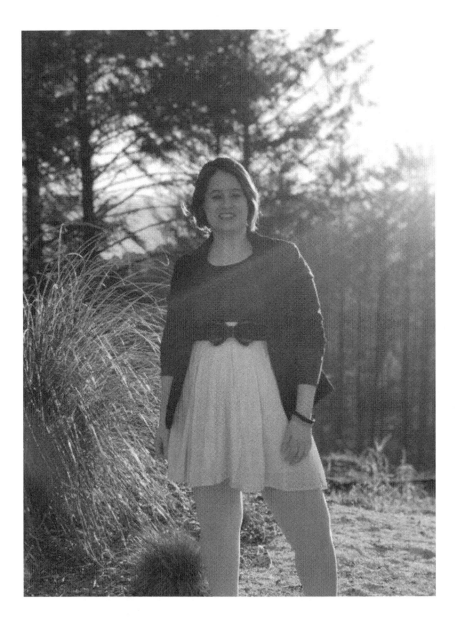

It Takes a Village

By Sarah Blackburn

My relationship with Mental health has been a leading role in my life since my teens. I was born in 1982 in Vancouver, Washington. The third daughter of my mother's third marriage. Or was it 4th? We lived in Spokane with my two brothers, two sisters and my father who sold advertising as a radio host when he wasn't running for president. Obviously that didn't pan out, and he started growing marijuana in the basement. After years of picking berries with her kids and an infant strapped to her, my mother left when she was pregnant with my brother. When he was just three months old, my father kidnapped all seven of us for three weeks. My mother has told me this story many times. About how the police wouldn't help her because she didn't have a custody order. How her milk dried up because her baby was gone. She couldn't eat or sleep. When she did get a court order and the police retrieved us, we all made reports of abuse against her and my stepfather. I can only remember bits and pieces of this whole event. Brief moments, like leaving in the police car as my younger sister cried and cried. I recall the police station and the carpet in the special room with toys. They gave me a teddy bear. I was so worried about my baby brother. He had trouble breathing, cried a lot, looked sick and wasn't really growing.

My father believed that he was rescuing us from a dangerous environment. He believed my mother and stepfather were horribly abusive to all of us. My mother was granted full custody after this incident. It was obvious to authorities that our stories were fake because we all used the exact same words. Line for line our claims of neglect and abuse were identical. Our words were dismissed. What they didn't know was that my mother and stepfather were incredibly volatile. It wasn't until I became an adult, I learned that domestic violence was their way of life. I thought the screaming and yelling was normal. I'll never forget my stepfather grabbing my mother by the throat and pushing her over the coach. That marriage ended shortly after another sibling joined our family.

In 1993, mom decided to relocate the four children she still had at home from Southern Central Oregon to NorthEast Arkansas. She claimed she wanted to be closer to her father, our grandfather. It was a long time before I learned the real reason we moved across the country. You see my father maintained that my mother was abusing us. He truly believed he needed to save us from her. He even wrote a book about this fantasy to set sail on the ocean with his children. Her father falling ill led us to visit the state of Arkansas and six months later, she moved us out there! My mother had finally found her power after starting college and was able to transfer to Arkansas State University where she would graduate in 1996 as a single mother of eight children.

On my 13th birthday, my father surprised us all by showing up in Arkansas. This was three months after hanging up on me during one of our weekly phone calls. During this call, I had interrupted him while I stood on his soapbox of judgement. I had finally demanded he stop lying about my mother and stepfather. Even though he was no longer in our lives, I had amazing memories of my stepfather being a real hands on Dad to me. Fishing trips to the coast, hiking, camping, crabbing,…. So many amazing memories. What I didn't have were memories of beatings, or being hungry, or sleeping with animals. Things were violent and angry between he and my mother, but the home I had when they were together had proper beds, and we received adequate care most of the time.

When my father disconnected the phone line, I realized that I was not the girl he thought I was. In that moment I realized he had told me so many things about myself and my life that weren't true. When he showed up on my birthday months later, I did not feel excited.

It was soon after that migraines began consuming my daily life. The migraines led to doctor's appointments, MRI's, and a lot of different medication trial and errors. I'd guess I was way overmedicated. I know I was experiencing hallucinations. I remember once seeing a stuffed teddy bear stand up in my brothers' room, wave and sit back down. I hid under the covers until my local b.f.f. Zach showed up to hang out with me.

Self Care Sarah developed after years of Sad Sarah, Suicidal Sarah, and Self Harm Sarah running the show. Mental health for me is all about checking in with myself. Becoming aware of my physical and emotional being or Self Assessing is something I do it a lot. I ask myself questions like "How am I doing right now? How do I feel in this moment? Can I give my emotions names? How does my physical body feel?" The physical assessment helps me identify where i'm holding tension whether from the joints in my fingers or the muscles in my neck, glutes or feet. Tensing and relaxing is something I started doing after I took Bradley ChildBirth classes during my pregnancy with my son. The instructor had such a beautiful air about her. We got to meet her lovely husband and their 4 kids including a nursling during the weeks of the course she taught from her in-laws very nice home in East Salem. I so vividly remember the experience. I felt so connected to my then husband and in touch with myself, and our growing baby.

For me, managing my mental health is more than just my physical body.

My wellness has always been hinged on community. My belief is that I need human connection to be healthy.

I want to tell you the story of Sad Sarah who tried to kill herself during winter break 96'-97' of her freshman year of high school.

We lived on Kimberly Road.. or was it st? In Paragould Arkansas in a three bedroom two bath one level home. It was made of brick and had a giant tree in the front. It had a carport and a fenced back yard. I used to climb on the roof all the time. I was such a tomboy. My best friend and I bonded for the first time racing bikes my very first day on the block. It was a decent neighborhood with a lot of other kids. One family had a sweet pool we got invited too pretty often. That family and my besties had quads that we all got to ride around on. There was a huge open field next to a forest just 2 blocks over that we loved zipping around through the snow dragging a tire behind us. That was our idea of fun as a young teenager growing up in the south.

My mom was single at the time and attending ASU about half an hour away. That meant five days a week plus two to four nights she would stay and go to the bar, we were home alone. I remember having chore instructions and dinner directions. Very basic stuff like, sweep and mop, laundry, help the boys clean up their room.

Being five of eight, I was the oldest of the kids left at home. I was responsible for my three younger siblings when she was gone.

My oldest sister went to college and then into the airforce!
My oldest brother was incarcerated and then disappeared.

My second oldest sister lived with our Father.

My second oldest brother was in a detention center.

So I was the babysitter which I could totally handle at 14. When this incident occurred, I was 14, Penny 12, Ben, 9 Thomas 7

On Friday nights, I got a coke and a bag of pretzels as babysitting payment.

Penny usually took off with her friends. Ben and Thomas hung out with neighbor kids and basically did their own thing. My only job was to feed them and get them to bed. Ben was the absolute worst at night. He would terrorize Thomas and when I'd attempt to put him in time out his response would be to climb out the window and run down the street. I can remember feeling so embarrassed that people must think I was hurting him as he ran away screaming.

This routine worked until it didn't. In the fall of my freshman year, I began having migraines and insomnia. My mom took me to the doctor many times. However, my symptoms of nausea, sensitivity to light, and pain never went away no matter how many different combinations we tried.

I was falling dramatically behind in school and had completely isolated myself from my best friend network. I have never been a big crowd person. Even in high school, I had 2 or 3 besties. During this time, I completely cut them out.

What I haven't mentioned is the violence that existed in our home. My younger sister was lashing out over everything and anything. She became irate and stabbed me in the back with a pencil when I denied her my favorite shirt. I remember it had the word POLO embroidered on it. Back in the days of ZCavaricci and Guess being THE COOLESTS brands! How about L.A. Gear shoes? Ahhh those were the days.

This story is hard for me to tell. I hope you'll pardon my brevity. I want to share this because the things I believed when I was suicidal weren't real. They were stories. Learning to tell the difference between what actually happened and what I made it mean about myself has been my biggest transformation.

Being physically attacked seemed to be something that was happening on a constant basis. Whether it was my mom aggressively parenting, my younger brother rebelling, or my sister bullying, physical abuse was part of our day to day lifestyle. What broke me that day was verbal abuse. After months at home having isolated myself from my friend circle, I had begun to believe the words of hate being spewed at me. I believed no one loved me. I believed I was unwanted. I believed I was a waste of space.

There is this running joke in my family that I am the milk man's and not my father's. I don't know if it's because I have brown hair and not blonde like my sisters, but my mother swears there was no milk man.

Which I really don't see why the different parentage mattered so much. Of the 8 of us, there are 4 fathers. My father and Mother had 5 children together. My mother had 2 children previously from 2 different marriages. My mother had another marriage and child after her divorce from my father. 2 marriages in fact.

My father had a wife and daughter before my mother. I guess I should be saying that I am 6 of 9 instead of 5 of 8? I have never believed in differentiating between step/half/whole siblings. I believe siblings are siblings and the extra words can be used when it's necessary to make a distinction.

But is it necessary?
Is making the distinction necessary?
Just something I ponder as we introduce ourselves to the world.
You see.. I , Like my mother.. Have children from 4 men.

But that's another story.

This story is about the day I took every single pill in the medicine cabinet in my mom's bathroom while she was at work. More than 300 when combined with all the tried and failed prescriptions i'd been put on over the past 6 months to treat my migraines and insomnia.

Penny and I had been in a verbal altercation for what felt like hours. I was hearing how I should not exist because I have no friends, I'm ugly, I'm disgusting, I smell bad, my hair is greasy, no one likes me, no one wants me, basically how worthless to society I am. The verbal abuse occurred, and I made it mean that those things were true of me. I created a reality based on the abuse in which I believed my family would be better off if I didn't exist. Now, as a healed adult. I take responsibility for creating that reality. I made those words mean things about myself instead of identifying them as verbal abuse. I am whole, perfect, and complete exactly as I am.

I went to my mom's bathroom. A tiny closet of a space. I stood staring at myself in the mirror as I took handful after handful of Gelcaps, powder coats, mostly small ones, pills in between sips of water. To this day, I cannot even take a tylenol without causing my gag reflex to kick in.

I went into the living room and dumped the empty bottles in front of my sister and said "You win.". I went back to my mom's room and got into her bed and fell asleep.

It was winter break. My mom was at work for the day. According to my Mom, when she got home from work, Penny said that I had a migraine and took a pill to go to sleep. Mom let me sleep. She climbed into bed with me that night and got up and went to work the next day. Upon coming home from work on her lunch break to find me still in bed asleep, she panicked.

I can remember her trying to get me in the shower and my legs not working. Trying to speak was almost impossible because everything was garbled. I don't remember the trip to the hospital. I don't remember checking in. I don't remember the next day. I was told that it had been too long since I'd ingested the pills to pump my stomach. I have broken bits of memory. My dad came to visit. My brother's girlfriend was there at some point too. I recall picking white fluffies off her jeans and handing them to her. I was hallucinating. Much of my hospital stay was a blur. I know I was not allowed to go home. My sister Christine and her husband who were currently stationed on Keesler Airforce base in Gulfport Mississippi offered to take me in. When I was released from the hospital, I stayed with my sister Elizabeth, her husband Michael and their baby Tristan in January 97 for a few days until my eldest sister Christine could get a few days leave to pick me up.

I moved in with her for the second half of my Freshman year. I never went to counseling. I told people I needed space and that I was recovering from trauma. I wore black all the time. I did a lot of staring off into space and rocking back and forth while listening to KoRn (heavy metal) as loud as it would go on my brother-in-laws stereo. That semester of school taught me a lot about the world I didn't know, but that's another story.

I have never again allowed myself to feel so alone. At 37 years old, I have learned to recognize the signs of my anxiety, manic depression, and panic disorder. Recognizing the signs, being aware of how I'm doing has empowered me to take responsibility for my own mental health.

I one had it described to me as a quilt.

For me to be mentally healthy, I need to be connected to my village. My village, or quilt is made up of a mental health care professional, a counselor, my primary care physician, I am a member of overeaters anonymous. I go to a yoga class once a week. I have been going to the same gym for more than 10 years. I am part of many online organizations. I keep in touch with old friends. I make new friends. And for me, I am and will always be enrolled in some sort of educational training.

I'm currently in a program called The Self Expression Leadership Program which is part of Landmark. My next step is to get certified in neuro linguistic programming through a company called Manifest Destiny. By fall of 2020, I will be enrolled in community college.

You see, I've built a life that includes activities and people that support the lifestyle that works best for me. I truly believe in a healthy, active lifestyle that is centered around education. I cannot imagine a better life for my children. A life in which they are aware of mental health, but it does not run our lives.

I'd like to leave you with strong encouragement to go create a quilt that works for you. Reach out to your village and see where you can be strong and where you need support. Recovery for me means staying connected.

Acknowledgements

I'd like to take a moment to acknowledge all the teachers, leaders, counselors, and mentors who believed in me when I did not. As a junior in high school, teachers sent home class work for me to do when I was home for 6 weeks with my daughter. I was given access to the nurse's office to pump so that I could maintain the breastfeeding relationship.

There was even a work program that allowed me to be present with my daughter in her daycare while giving me the skills I needed to be a present, hands on mom. I have felt the most empowered when being directed towards resources rather than being labeled as "low income", "needy", or as a "survivor". It was only when I took responsibility for my own well being that I was able to make strong connections to those who could stand with me in that possibility.

About Sarah Blackburn

Sarah Blackburn is a wife and mother of six. She lives on the beautiful Central Oregon Coast with husband Adam, all six children, three cats, two dogs, and a very questionable tank of sea monkeys. She works from home as a social media marketing consultant and website designer for her company The Power Parents Online Community. Sarah is passionate about serving parents who want to learn how to financially support their families while being physically present.

At age 14, Sarah was hospitalized for overdosing on prescription medications. While this was her only attempt to end her life, self-harm became a part of her everyday existence until age 32.

As a "Teen Mom All Grown Up" Sarah advocates strongly for self-love and self-care. Her passion inspired her to create a Facebook community that has evolved over the past three years into a place for women to practice radical acceptance, unconditional love, and to begin to explore what healing looks like for them. This community uses tools such as breath work, meditation, visualization, spoken affirmations, keeping a gratitude journal, stream of consciousness writing activities, and consuming personal development content as well as nutritional supplements, essential oils, CBD, cannabis, and seeking professional help. If we believe it takes a village to raise a child, then I invite you to consider it takes a village to support a mother.

Made in the
USA
Lexington, KY